Dr. Bach's
Flower Remedies

tapping into the positive emotional qualities of the chakras

Philip Salmon and Anna Jeoffroy

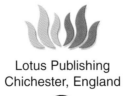

Lotus Publishing
Chichester, England

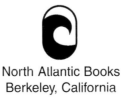

North Atlantic Books
Berkeley, California

First published in 1998 by Energy Works (0 9528044 2 5).
This edition published in 2006 by
Lotus Publishing
3. Chapel Street, Chichester, PO19 1BU and
North Atlantic Books
P O Box 12327
Berkeley, California 94712

Publisher's Note

The contents of this book are the opinions of the authors based on their experience, research, and interests. It is designed for reference purposes only, and to stimulate further research into flower and other essences. It is not in any way a substitute for a properly qualified, professional healthcare practitioner. Any person with a condition requiring medical attention should consult a medical practitioner. Neither the authors, nor the publisher, can promise or accept responsibility for the efficacy of the remedies.

Acknowledgements

Many thanks to Adrian Jameson whose horticultural expertise has been an inspiration.

Drawings Wal Provost
Text and Cover Design Wendy Craig
Printed and Bound in the UK by Scotprint

Dr. Bach's Flower Remedies: tapping into the positive emotional qualities of the chakras is sponsored by the Society for the Study of Native Arts and Sciences, a nonprofit educational corporation whose goals are to develop an educational and cross-cultural perspective linking various scientific, social, and artistic fields; to nurture a holistic view of arts, sciences, humanities, and healing; and to publish and distribute literature on the relationship of mind, body, and nature.

British Library Cataloguing in Publication Data

A CIP record for this book is available from the British Library
ISBN 1 905367 04 X (Lotus Publishing)
ISBN 1 55643 640 8 (North Atlantic Books)

Library of Congress Cataloguing-in-Publication Data

Salmon, Philip.
  [Dr. Bach's flower remedies and the chakras]
  Dr. Bach's flower remedies : tapping into the positive emotional qualities
of the chakras / Philip Salmon and Anna Jeoffroy.
     p. ; cm.
  Originally published as: Dr. Bach's flower remedies and the chakras.
  Includes bibliographical references.
  ISBN-10: 1-905367-04-X (pbk.)
  ISBN-13: 978-1-55643-640-6 (NAB : pbk.)
  ISBN-10: 1-55643-640-8 (NAB : pbk.)
  1. Flowers--Therapeutic use. 2. Chakras. I. Jeoffroy, Anna. II. Title.
III. Title: Flower remedies. IV. Title: Doctor Bach's flower remedies.
  [DNLM: 1. Bach, Edward, 1886-1936. 2. Medicine, Herbal. WB 925 S172d
2006]
RX615.F55S25 2006
615'.321--dc22
                    2006025968

Contents

Introduction

Philip Salmon came across the Bach Remedies 30 years ago whilst working at Enton Hall Natural Health Clinic. Anna Jeoffroy began to use them 16 years ago, around the time she began to practice as a professional reflexologist.

They both worked with them as part of the journal keeping segment of a self-development module for students whom they trained on Philip Salmon's reflexology course. They gained deeper insights into the remedies whilst working with students in class over a 3 to 4 year period. The probing questions asked by students required a much more thorough investigation into exactly how the remedies worked.

From his knowledge of Colour Therapy, Philip realised that the colours allocated by Dr. Bach to the seven groups into which he had divided his remedies broadly related to the rainbow colours of the chakras. Whilst working more intensely with this insight, Philip and Anna developed the ideas to the point where they realised that the positive qualities of the remedies relate to the positive qualities of the chakras. They then developed the ideas until they could be presented as a workshop to other practitioners.

They offer their understanding of the flower remedies in relation to the chakras to enhance the general understanding of the Bach remedies – not to supersede or replace anything. There are many well-trained professional practitioners, or those who have worked with the remedies for years, who have accurate ways of identifying the appropriate remedy for use by a patient. They may find this book gives them a further tool at their disposal. Many more people who are interested in the remedies may find self-diagnosis a little daunting in the light of so many remedies, especially if there is not an obvious one for the problem. It is accepted by energy practitioners working on the body that the body itself does not lie: reflexologists, kinesiologists, shiatsu practitioners, and acupuncturists will all refer to the body to diagnose areas of imbalance, preferring this information to that proffered by the client, if they differ. On this basis, identifying a chakra area that is manifesting imbalance at a physical level can quickly help us to get to the source of the problem.

Although Dr. Bach worked intuitively to discover the remedies, the authors feel confident from reading numerous of his published works that Dr. Bach knew that he was placing the remedies into groups related to the chakras. In placing them into seven groups he then allocated colours that relate almost exactly to the rainbow colours of the chakras. This method of working with the chakras makes the remedies so easy to understand, it seems clear that he knew exactly what he was doing.

This technique, along with working towards the positive qualities of the chakra system as opposed to focusing on the negative state, enables us to derive the maximum benefit from these wonderful remedies.

Those who have attended the workshop on which this book is based have found that working with the remedies in relation to the chakras enables very clear insights into which remedy or remedies might be the most appropriate for any condition.

How to Use This Book

Edward Bach was a medical doctor, qualified surgeon, held a diploma in Public Health and was a highly regarded medical researcher. Inevitably in anyone coming from this background when discussing disease he focused on the negative condition to be cleared. Indeed in *The Medical World* in 1930 he wrote that, "as healers we must focus on the negatives to be cured". Yet when discussing the enlivening effect or influence of flowers and as we believe the chakras, he also knew that no improvement in the human condition or health was possible without an opening and atunement to the higher chakras. An 'opening to the virtues' as Dr. Bach said.

In working towards the virtues, flower remedies are an ideal tool to work with from a self-development point of view as they will help people to work with, and clear emotional blocks to their development. This is a working towards the virtues in Dr. Bach's terminology.

To enable this book to be used by both those interested in healing and those who wish to work on their own development, the heading 'Negative State' is worded from the point of view of those interested in healing, and the heading 'The Action of the Remedy', is worded from the point of view of those interested in working on their own (or with others) self-development.

Each Chakra group begins with a page that explains the general qualities of the Chakra. The age range when the qualities of that Chakra predominate in our life and the remedies in that group.

In the double page spread on each remedy, the left-hand page shows a sketch of the flower/tree/water from which the remedy is made. The qualities or energy signature which we believe indicates why this flower/tree/water was chosen to make a remedy.

In 'Chakra Qualities' we indicate which aspect of the Chakra energy is being affected by the remedy.

In 'Positive Qualities', we indicate the positive or 'virtuous' state that the remedy works towards. This is worth bearing in mind when trying to identify a remedy for someone: it is more comfortable for them to see that they want to feel more secure and independent than to suggest that they are clingy and dependent. When we work towards the positive we automatically and painlessly allow the negative to dissolve. This applies in both the therapy and the self-development situation.

The 'Negative State' and 'The Action of the Remedy' are dealt with above.

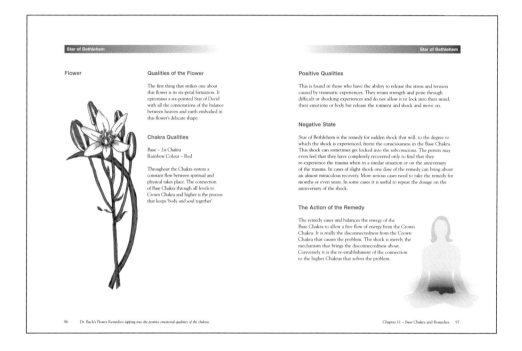

CHAPTER 1

Edward Bach

Edward Bach was born in 1886, and died in 1936. He was a medical doctor and researcher (bacteriologist), who became dissatisfied with the medical orthodoxy of his time. He developed his own system of treating illness based on the healing properties of flowers.

Then as indeed up to the present day, medical orthodoxy held that germs or viruses cause disease. Bach became convinced from his research as a bacteriologist as well as from the practical clinical experience he gained from seeing patients, that germs would not gain a foothold and grow in the body unless the ground had been prepared first.

Bach realised that the 'ground' was largely prepared by the mind. If a person was balanced, optimistic, outgoing and positive in life, then the vital energies that created that person would flow unhindered, creating vital good health. This is not health, which is a mere absence of pain and a body that functions, but a vibrant overflowing good health.

If on the other hand the person was pessimistic, insular and negative, these mental and emotional states would inhibit or block the flow of vital energy. This would create stagnant areas in the body, which would become depleted so that they would be ideal breeding grounds for bacteria thereby enabling them to gain a foothold, and break down the tissues causing disease. These observations and beliefs fit perfectly with the holistic view of health, which is that all aspects of each individual's personality, psyche and emotional state have consequences at the physical level.

Many scientists are now beginning to accept that the energy patterns of the universe are somehow connected with our life force patterns, and that all energy emanates from one original source.

Throughout our being, are repeating patterns – they repeat throughout the physical body – eyes, ears, face, hands, feet, even our cells, but they also interpenetrate the layers of our emotional, psychological and spiritual being.

When distortions occur within a layer of energy, the pattern is distorted, then what we would recognise as a negative pattern is allowed to dominate. This will alter the individual's ability to follow their true path and achieve their full potential. The remedies enable the energy system to re-pattern, by introducing it to a positive pattern, which stimulates the distortions and damage to be transformed, rebalanced and harmonised.

CHAPTER 2

The Journey of Consciousness Through the Body

The energy that creates us and gives us life, originates in pure spirit. Whilst this vital energy flows freely through our body, we have good health. If there is an impediment or a block to the flow of this vital energy, we have disease and ultimately, death. The flow of this energy is sometimes referred to as 'the journey of consciousness through the body'.

Consciousness originates in a region of pure spirit. In this state it is pure unconditional love, totally connected to and at one with all that exists. In order to gain wisdom by learning from experience it takes on limitations and forgets its divine origin. This is what we experience when we come into matter.

As consciousness descends into matter, it 'goes to sleep' losing all awareness of its divine origin. On the return journey it evolves into spirit and 'wakes up' becoming conscious once again of its divinity. The two forces we work with in this world are a drive to wake up and a falling back into unconsciousness.

Consciousness comes into the body through the Crown Chakra, travels down through the centre of the spinal cord and grounds itself in the material world through the Base Chakra. It then travels back up through the body to the Crown Chakra and back into the realm of the spirit.

If this journey through the body is unhindered, the spirit (which is consciousness) achieves its purpose, which is to gain wisdom. On the other hand, if the flow is blocked for any reason, then the resulting blockage manifests as chaos within the body. This is experienced as physical disease and mental illness, precisely the conditions that the remedies are designed to counter.

Our negative emotional states interfere with the flow of consciousness. The Bach remedies help to raise our vibration, thereby lifting our spirits back to a positive state. This will clear the blockage allowing the energy to flow freely again, thereby restoring vibrant good health.

The positive qualities of the seven groups of remedies are related to the positive qualities of the seven major chakras in the body. The positive qualities of the remedies clear blockages in the chakras, thereby ensuring an unhindered flow of vital conscious energy through the body.

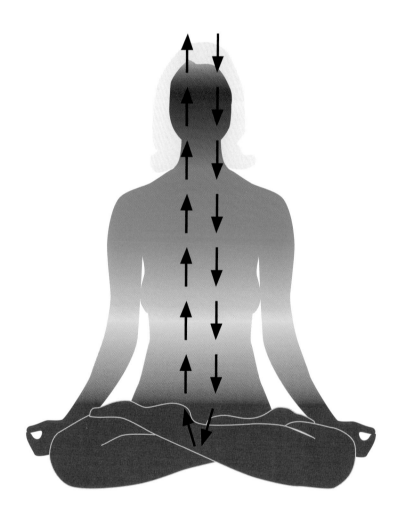

Scientists measure energy in many ways using a variety of different 'meters'. Decibel meters are used to measure sound, photon counters to measure light and voltmeters to measure electricity and so on. All scientifically recognised forms of energy have appropriate measuring systems and devices. These devices are not yet available to measure all the levels of energy that we experience in and around us. Many people are sensitive to these energies and can identify differing speeds of vibration in other peoples' energy because they can feel these vibrations. They do this within their own energy bodies, and then interpret what they feel, using their body's tools of touch, vision and sometimes hearing. If they use sight they can then 'see' different vibratory levels within the chakras as colours. The highest vibration is at the Crown Chakra that can often appear to have a violet light around it, and then as the vibration decreases in steps through the different chakras, it creates a subtle change observable through the rainbow colours as follows:

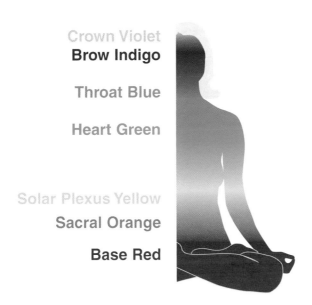

At each step down there is a slowing of the vibration that is 'seen' as a change in colour. This description of the chakra colours is inevitably simplistic. It is not meant to be literally true. Each chakra has all energy vibrations within it but certain frequencies predominate at each level from the Crown Chakra down to the Base Chakra. These are described by using the rainbow colours as our measuring devise because it colours closely represent the differing energy at each chakra level.

CHAPTER 3

Chakras and Physical / Emotional / Mental Development

The simplest way to get to grips with the creation of the body through the chakra system is to start at the beginning, with the ovum and the sperm.

At the point of conception a double vortex is created, which is connected by a cord. The top vortex becomes the Crown Chakra and the lower vortex the Base Chakra. The connecting cord is the spinal cord. The vibratory levels that become the other chakras spin out from the spinal cord. This all happens simultaneously, not one at a time, like the unfolding of a leaf as it grows.

Although the different levels of energy come into existence at the same time and all are, to some extent, active the whole time, some are more active than others at different times of life. The more active phases of these cycles are known as the 'Seven Ages of Man'.

It is important to be clear that we all work through these energies in our own way and at our own speed. We can, for a variety of reasons, become blocked at any level, or by suffering shock or trauma regress to a childish level. The Bach remedies are extremely useful, enabling us to clear blockages and move on to the next level of wisdom. The chakras create the physical, emotional, mental and spiritual bodies. Releasing old self-defeating patterns of energy from any chakra, not only increases wisdom and knowing but also improves mental, emotional and spiritual health.

1st age: from birth to about seven years of age the Base chakra energies of survival, drive, and the will to be in the world are our predominant energies.

At this stage our whole life revolves around 'Me'. Do I have food, water, and warmth? Until about three years of age we have little concept of anything else: if someone is with us they exist, but if they are not, they cease to be.

2nd age: from 7 to 14 years as the emotional, Sacral Chakra energies come more into play, we become aware of relationships with others, of how they effect us. We are establishing our ability to 'trade' as in, you give me friendship and I will be your friend too. We begin to think slightly less of self and begin to move out into the world and relate to others. Our best friend in the whole world is most important to us at this stage in our development. It is an age when shock and trauma to the emotional system can impair our ability to relate to people, or to be able to 'give and take' in a relationship in future years.

3rd age: from 14 to 21 years the Solar Plexus Chakra energies begin to predominate. The teenage years are a time when we begin to establish ourselves as individuals in the world. It is important to have a sense of belonging: to be accepted as part of the group or 'gang'. We begin to mark out our territory, decide what our future will be, and move out into and begin to try to make some sense of the world. It is at this stage we begin to set our career path and feel a direction for our future. Traditionally it is at 21 years of age when a person becomes an adult. By this time, the lower three material and self-centred chakras have been worked through, and the young person begins to transform into an adult.

4th age: from 21 to 28 years of age the Heart Chakra energies come more into play. This is the time when people begin to open up to each other much more, get married and bring children into the world. At this time of life the energies are transforming from self and the needs of self to taking others into one's heart, and being deeply concerned about their needs to the extent that we are prepared to put these needs before our own. This is the level where we connect with unconditional love, which must be understood refers to accepting others for what they are: not for being servile and living as a victim. These are the qualities needed to be in a successful relationship and parenting.

5th age: from 28 to 35 are times of communication and healing. Healing in this sense is about bringing people and ideas together with sufficient harmony and organisation (communication) so that things can grow and develop. It is often a time of intense progress within one's career, where the elements of life are brought together, fused and allowed to grow into new forms. This is a time when sometimes, quite spontaneously, negative patterns within our etheric blueprint begin to readjust as we connect with our higher self and therefore our true-life path.

6th age: from 35 to 42 the higher mental energies begin to come into play. This is often a time of inner crises, relationship problems and questions such as: "Who am I?", "Why am I doing this?", "What is it all about?" and, "What does it matter anyway?". In an attempt to resolve these issues, people will often begin to look for a perfect career, relationship, lifestyle; or make adjustments within their existing lifestyle to bring it closer to their idea of perfection. This is a necessary but impossible quest at this level of existence, but much more is learned about oneself in the attempt.

7th age: from 42 to 49 is the time when, traditionally, transpersonal and universal concerns come more to the fore in life. By now, concerns have moved on from the self, through friendships and permanent relationships to the family, the extended family and the tribe, then onto the wider community and the country. Now the issues are becoming global and universal. Man and his place in the cosmos, rather than, just me in my world. If these are faced and resolved successfully, then a time of greater security and wisdom come into life.

At age 49 we begin the cycle again, but from a higher point on the spiral and with the benefit of past experience. At this age, the material becomes important again as people begin to reassess their lives and themselves. This age reflects similar qualities to the original Base chakra energy. It is more concerned with what we have achieved, making serious provision for old age, or having acquired a good standard of living, beginning to recognise that there is more to our existence than merely the pointless acquisition of wealth.

At 56 the energy that comes into play is again about relationships. We often find ourselves building new relationships and friendships with people in whose company we feel at ease. We no longer feel it necessary to prove ourselves, and we are more accepting of others and ourselves.

At 63 we come again to the Solar Plexus energy. This time the issues are about our independence or perhaps our inter dependence. We may look for a direction as we traditionally approach or begin retirement. This is a time many people find difficult as they have their financial independence, purpose and direction in life taken from them.

A further transformation, moving once again to another level of connection to the more spiritual energies, takes place from 70 with heart felt love and acceptance.

Communication and healing again comes into its own from about 77. The wise man or woman of the community is able to see things from a higher perspective, helping to hold the pattern of the throat energy, facilitating change within a community. Our elders are in the main no longer respected and revered as elders with wisdom and guidance to share. This perhaps accounts for the fact that many of them retreat into fragile worlds of their own from this age, beginning to show a vastly reduced interest in the world at large. By turning deeper within, they avoid their disenchantment with the world around them, unfortunately thereby depriving the world of the benefit of their wisdom.

The connection with the spiritual energies strengthens further through the ages of 84 and 91 taking us to the third set of cycles that start at 98 years of age: then so on in seven-year cycles.

This map of energy cycles should be thought of as an ebb and flow of energy as, say, represented on a weather forecast chart, where many influences can affect the final outcome, rather than a time chart where one thing happens rigidly after another. The chakra energies not only create the body but are also stages of learning that we grow through, and inevitably we work through all of them at the same time. Although age is a useful marker as to which energy will predominate, many factors can bring it in early or delay it until later in life. In the same way that certain conditions will cause the physical body to mature more quickly or block our development. But the stages of development must be worked through in a certain order; for instance, we cannot be adults before we are children, nor do we run before we have learned how to walk. Our success at each previous stage will determine how far we can develop in the next stage.

CHAPTER 4

Balancing Positive and Negative

A lifestyle, an opinion, an emotion, a chakra, indeed any facet of our life or being can be out of balance. It may be too far one way or another, too outgoing or too introverted, too open, or too closed. There is a magical middle way or balance that allows great sweeps of energy movement, like a man and a woman dancing, but never loses its rhythm. We should be able to be wide open when it is appropriate and also able to close down when it is prudent to do so. Whether we feel we are walking a tightrope or riding a motorcycle across country, we seek the balance of action not of rigidity.

Without this ability to move we become rigid: rigidity is death, rigor mortis and eventually dust. Our life, our dreams our relationships and our ambitions can end in this way, if through fear, inertia, and dullness of mind or lack of ambition we do not act. On the other hand if we rush around trying to make everything right, constantly interfere or nag others, keep pulling the plant up to check that the roots are developing well, we risk destroying the very thing we are trying to accomplish.

The challenge is to find our way through by taking appropriate action, not too much not too little, the action appropriate to the challenge whether that challenge is dancing or walking a tightrope.

Every part of our being vibrates at certain frequencies. Sometimes through shock, unbalanced lifestyle and emotional trauma's these vibrations become too sharp or too flat, and we become like a musical note that is slightly off key. When we are looking at the positive qualities in the remedies, we are looking for dynamic balance.

To resolve the problem we must offer the true 'note' to the body so that it can use it as a tuning fork to restore the perfect vibration and thereby re-establish balance.

The primary energy flow through our being is through the chakras. They react and respond to our environment and the circumstances of our life continually. When we are relaxed and happy they will be open, when we feel threatened at any level of our being, our chakras close, drawing our energy closer to us. This is a normal and protective response to different kinds of stimulus. If this did not happen, we would not be able to respond appropriately to anything or anybody. Through imbalance, the chakra energy may become too open, leaving us vulnerable to absorbing negativity that we should avoid. Alternatively, if this energy is restricted we are unable to open ourselves to normal healthy interaction with everything around us. This then has an effect at every level of our being, from our emotional state to our mental and eventually physical wellbeing.

The remedies work by normalizing vibrations, allowing the energies of the physical and subtle bodies to flow without resistance. This enables us to be able to respond appropriately in all circumstances.

Each chakra works independently, as well as working in harmony with each other. Although it is good to ensure they are all able to be responsive, we need to learn the art of observing their reactions rather than controlling them. As with the use of the breath of relaxation, we should not seek to control, but simply to observe. If we are always pre-empting our chakra energy, we disconnect ourselves from our divine source of information. We override the natural instincts of our chakras to respond intuitively. Anyway, we have enough to do without having to open and close our chakras in the same way that we have no need to take on the conscious responsibility for breathing in and out.

As we look at Dr. Bach's flower remedies in their seven groups, relating them to the chakras, we see how they allow us to fine-tune the different vibratory levels of the chakra qualities. These qualities are like strands of our emotions weaving together. Where one or another strand is too tight or too loose it affects not only the whole chakra, but will have a knock on effect on the rest of the system and the whole person.

Some people find it difficult to identify the appropriate emotion and therefore the ideal remedy to take. By recognizing the connection between remedy groups and chakras, we can identify the emotion through the area of the body that manifest disorder, thereby pinpointing for us the band of frequencies that needs addressing, helping us to choose a remedy or remedies that will bring us towards dynamic balance.

Working in this way with the remedies also encourages us to look and work towards the positive outcomes we desire, as opposed to focusing our energy on the negative state we may be in.

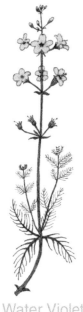

Water Violet
HOTTONIA palustris

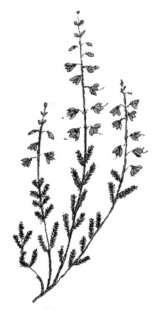

Heather
CALLUNA vulgaris

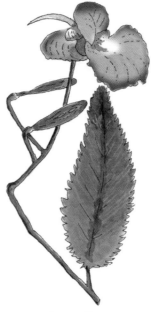

Impatiens
IMPATIENS royalei

CHAPTER 5

Crown Chakra and Remedies

Rainbow Colour Violet

Energy Quality – Pure Spirit
7th Age – From 42 Years to 49 Years

This transpersonal Chakra connects us to our divine nature, divine truth, and our spiritual being. Our spirit is connected to and interpenetrates the divine nature and spiritual being of all life. Concerns affecting the whole of creation are the field of action of this Chakra.

Disconnectedness manifests as loneliness, as in a person not connected to their source of being. We therefore close off from others, but in doing so, close off our connection to our source. Alternatively, we try to find a source outside ourselves, drawing on others for it or by dashing around searching for knowledge and wisdom. Of course the answers lie within ourselves, and through stillness and mediation we can reconnect with our truth, our path, and our universal consciousness or being.

Remedy Group
Loneliness

Remedies
Water Violet, Impatiens, Heather

The Flower

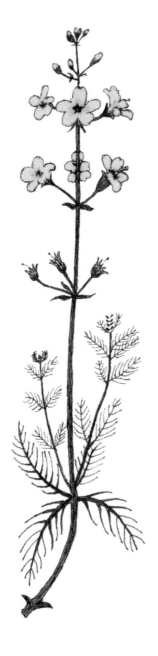

Qualities of the Flower

This flower begins life in the mud at the bottom of the pond and grows through the water. It will eventually emerge into air and sunlight to flower, thus transcending the limitations of the pond to be able to expand in all its glory, like the soul's journey from the dross of material life to spiritual enlightenment.

Chakra Qualities

Crown – *7th Chakra*
Rainbow Colour – Violet

Our spirit is connected to and interpenetrates the spiritual being of all life. Concerns affecting the whole of creation are the field of action of this Chakra. Disconnectedness manifests as the loneliness of a person who is not connected to universal love, wisdom and truth.

Positive Qualities

A connection to our divine nature gives us natural poise, grace and dignity. We have an inner certainty that we are never 'alone' even when we are enjoying periods of solitude. We have innate wisdom, which enables us to be wise counsellors. We know how to be helpful, what is often more important, and when to offer help. We are able to provide those around us with a safe and supportive environment in which to find resolution to problems or inner conflicts.

Negative State

Without this quality we stand aloof from others not realising that all beings have an inner connection. It is the aloofness of arrogance and lack of humility, which hardens the heart and leads to deep loneliness. It is often highly competent people who, because they deprive themselves of contact with others, even though it is by their own choice, become sullen, inward and overly defensive. When children are deprived of touch and contact with others they become introverted, sullen and fail to develop: all classic water violet characteristics.

The Action of the Remedy

The remedy helps to foster love for all, approachability and the general softening of a rigid personality. It will clear the blocks through the whole Chakra system allowing the lower energies to be revitalised and continue with their life task of transcending the physical back to spiritual energy.

The Flower

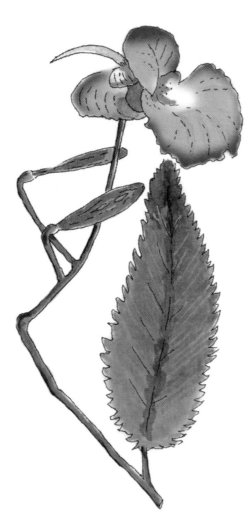

Qualities of the Flower

This plant grows profusely with divine poise and balance. The delicate pale flowers seem to float as if independent of time and space. It is a prolific plant that can overrun everything around it if not held in check. Where this happens, it demonstrates the chaos that can come from impatience.

Chakra Qualities

Crown – *7th Chakra*
Rainbow Colour – Violet

Because our spirit is connected to and interpenetrates the spiritual being of all life, when we are connected to it we automatically have a meaningful and loving connection to others. With this, we experience everything unfolding within the will of heaven and at the time which heaven dictates.

Positive Qualities

Those who from a deep intuitive knowing, give the will of heaven time and space to unfold. This gives them the patience, which is needed to allow right action time to grow into good outcomes. They also see the shortcomings of others as attempts to reach the truth, which simply need more time and patient endeavours to perfect.

Negative State

In this state, people feel that if only they can get their life sorted out, and also get those idiots who they work or live with to be more helpful, then everything will be fine. They fear that if they do not get things done now it will be too late and the opportunity will be gone forever. The disconnectedness manifests as a running around to sort things out rather than a connection to and trust in the divine.

The Action of the Remedy

The remedy helps to foster inner trust and calm. A sense that ultimately all beings are working together but at their own pace. There is no need to rush and push. Patience can accomplish more than irate rushing around and accomplish it even more quickly.

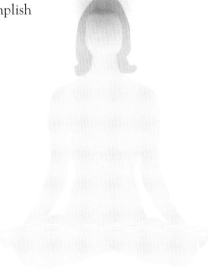

The Flower

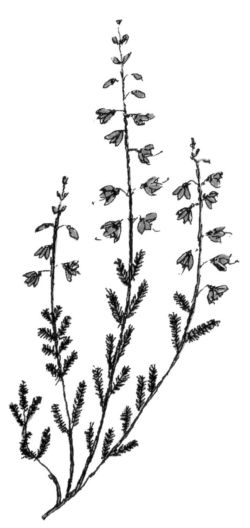

Qualities of the Flower

This plant has the ability to grow and thrive in the most rugged and inhospitable areas. It seems to have the ability to draw directly on universal energy for nourishment and strength.

Chakra Qualities

Crown – *7th Chakra*
Rainbow Colour – Violet

The spiritual being of the universe creates everything out of its own infinite energy. When we connect to it we have available to us the power which creates and sustains the universe. We help and support others by drawing on that strength. Lack of strength, love and vitality is a reminder to us that we have strayed from our source.

Positive Qualities

We can face any adversity that life presents to us because we draw our strength from the universe. When we can draw love and inspiration from the divine, adversity just melts away. By drawing our strength from the divine, we tap into the unlimited energy, which created the sun, the moon and the stars in the heavens, as well as every living being on earth. This abundant ever-flowing energy will effortlessly support us until the end of time.

Negative State

In this state we try to hide our loneliness, emptiness and fear by grabbing onto others for help and support and then draining them. We have all met people at a party who latch on to us, drone on at great length about themselves without letting us get a word in. When they have sucked us dry, they thank us for being such fascinating company then go off in search of another victim. They are like hungry ghosts who can only sustain themselves by draining others.

The Action of the Remedy

The remedy helps us to amplify our inner connection to the divine. It will engender an ambiance of peace, love and tranquillity at all times. This ultimately becomes our source of energy, power and strength in times of stress.

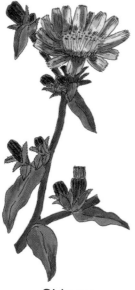

Chicory
CICHORIUM intybus

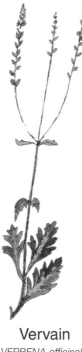

Vervain
VERBENA officinalis

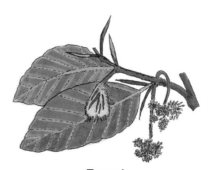

Beech
FAGUS sylvatica

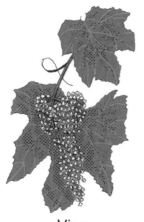

Vine
VITIS vinifera

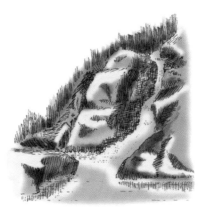

Rock Water

CHAPTER 6

Brow Chakra and Remedies
Rainbow Colour Indigo (Turquoise)

Energy Quality – Higher Mind/Spiritual
6th Age – From 35 Years to 42 Years

When you close your eyes and raise your attention to the Brow centre, you see darkness. This darkness is the colour of the sky at midnight. It is the final veil that separates the consciousness in the body from the higher spiritual worlds. It is sometimes referred to as the sky of the body. To pass through this darkness requires insight (to be able to see from within), intuition (to be able to accept tuition from within), and humility. These are the qualities needed to be able to find a way through, to a higher understanding of ourselves, and our purpose. Only faith and trust in the guidance given by our divine self enables us to progress. Inner reflection and meditation are the light and the path at this level. When we are disconnected we do not allow for insight and intuition, and all our energies are spent proving our worth by gaining knowledge to impress or influence others.

Remedy Group
Overcare for the welfare of others

Remedies
Chicory, Vervain, Beech, Vine, Rock Water

The Flower

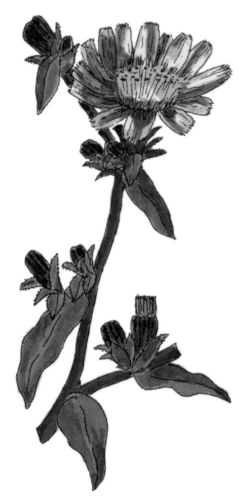

Qualities of the Flower

Giving totally of itself just for the joy of giving. Chicory flowers open each day in the knowledge that they are part of a greater plan. Each flower allows its neighbour the room to express its blossom. Chicory has a deep tap-root securing it firmly to the earth and the perseverance to keep flowering into late autumn when most other flowers have died off.

Chakra Qualities

Brow – *6th Chakra*
Rainbow Colour – Indigo

Insight and intuition are the qualities needed for development at this level, and an ability to trust one's own inner vision even though the way forward is not clear to the logical mind. This quality gives us the confidence to follow our own path, to be truly independent as in inner-dependence meaning a symbiotic relationship with everything within and around us, intuitively living in the flow of divine purpose.

Positive Qualities

We work from our centre of intuition, enabling us to give those around us appropriate support and the help they require, willingly and lovingly, whilst allowing them the space they need for their own growth and development.

Negative State

We are said to be in need of chicory when we demand attention the whole time. We are critical making demands of those around us, for instance the domineering mother with her children. The children's development is stunted by the domination of the parent and the parent's development is stunted because they are so busy sorting out their children's life that they pay no attention to their own development. The same quality can apply to anyone in a position of authority who tries to live their life through those around them.

The Action of the Remedy

The remedy helps us to loosen the reins and pay attention to our own growth and development. As we connect to our intuition we develop a sense of peace. This peace alleviates the incessant need to control and live everyone else's life for them. It brings out the 'good counsellor' in all of us, along with qualities of non-judgement and fairness allowing those around, the time and space to find their own intuitive path.

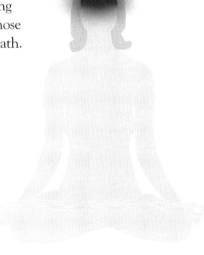

The Flower

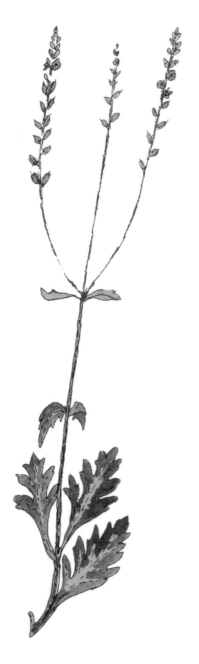

Qualities of the Flower

The demure flowers of this plant disguise its strength of character. Vervain has the strength and tenacity to grow in poor soil and waste ground without the need to make a big show of itself. It has a reputation for being helpful medicinally to protect against infection and cure disease and of having magical powers to ward off misfortune.

Chakra Qualities

Brow – *6th Chakra*
Rainbow Colour – Indigo

Quietness, reflection and tolerance are needed to remain in touch with the insight and intuition at the Brow centre. Key qualities at this level are the ability to be a good listener while maintaining one's own inner council.

Positive Qualities

Vervain brings the quality of clear sightedness, of being calm and steadfast in the face of adversity. To be able to follow our intuition (meaning listening to the teaching from within) helps us to trust our inner knowing and reach our goals irrespective of outer circumstances.

Negative State

Vervain is indicated for people who are forcefully opinionated, strong-willed and demanding. They need not only to be heard but that others agree with them. It is typical of those people who have been converted to a cause and are going to change the world, starting with you. These people have become arrogantly over enthusiastic, bullying and opinionated. In this state, they demand a soapbox and a large audience, unlike the chicory (previous remedy) who are happy to sound off from the dinner table.

The Action of the Remedy

The remedy promotes tolerance of the opinions of others. Helping us to realise that even when we are broadly right, other people can make a contribution that will lead to a more complete solution. The remedy re-establishes the equilibrium of inner steadfastness, outer love, service and tolerance.

The Tree

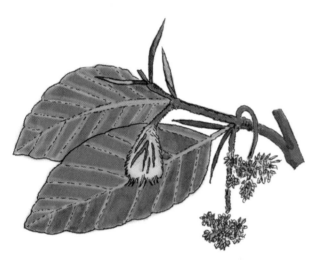

Qualities of the Tree

A solitary beech tree in a mixed wood best demonstrates the beech tree's positive qualities. It accepts other trees and growth around it whilst putting energy into its connection to its own life force through an abundance of foliage and deep secure roots. They are prolific and we often find woods being more and more taken over with beech. In a predominately beech wood, the overpowering energy of many trees together will thwart the growth of other trees and plants.

Chakra Qualities

Brow – *6th Chakra*
Rainbow Colour – Indigo

The quality is of accepting ourselves at a deep fundamental level allowing us to see ourselves as others see us. This enables us to accept the uniqueness and right to be, not only of ourselves but every other living thing.

Positive Qualities

We recognise our own worth and value, and we also see with clarity the value of allowing everyone to excel in their own way. We have a clear vision of other people that is tolerant and kind. We are secure in our own understanding of life's circumstances and are able to be great facilitators.

Negative State

The characteristics of this state are that we always find something to criticise and are never satisfied however much people try to be helpful. In this state, we have a tendency to be arrogant and bossy and see ourselves as so much more competent than others. A sour cynical approach to life creates inner tension because we are disconnected from our intuitive faculty. This inner tension causes us to project our intolerance of ourselves on to others.

The Action of the Remedy

The remedy softens arrogance, helping us to find our centre of truth within which leads us to a love and tolerance for ourselves, and a connection to the oneness of the universe. We are more understanding and able to accept that the faults of others are also part of our own being, not totally separate. This helps us to be more tolerant and helpful to those around us.

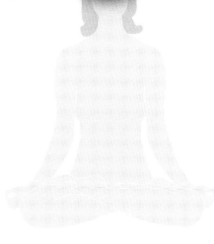

The Flower

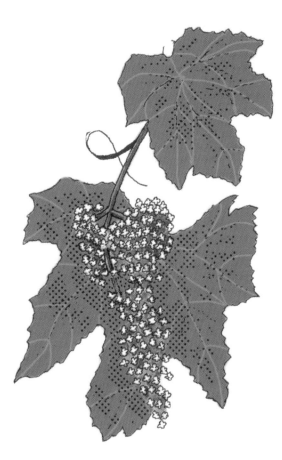

Qualities of the Flower

The vine plant will intuitively grow without fear or trepidation finding the support it needs at each stage to help it to climb higher. Flowering is not an attention seeking process, with the small flowers being displaced very quickly by the ripening stamens from which the grapes grow and ripen, allowing the vine to give generously of its fruit.

Chakra Qualities

Brow – *6th Chakra*
Rainbow Colour – Indigo

This quality allows a free flow of information (through intuition), releasing us from the need to hold on to old and rigid thought patterns, allowing us to progress freely along our path.

Positive Qualities

Connection to the intuitive centre of guidance and wisdom within helps us to develop as strong wise leaders. We lead not by force, but by guiding others to excel, progressing and performing at a higher level. We help to develop support networks for those around us. We are confident in our abilities to manage and are able to find any support needed, moving on from one stage to another easily. The action of this type of person is to climb to the top whilst nourishing everyone around them.

Negative State

This manifests as overbearing and dominating. People who climb to the top in their business or profession at great cost to their colleagues, with complete disregard for the needs of others, then use authority to dominate everyone. They are people who are so lost in the world that they fail to look within themselves. Their desperate need for success leads them to drive others to obtain the recognition they crave, rather than leading from their own inner guidance and wisdom. They can also become clingy, not trusting that as one focus leaves their life, another can come in.

The Action of the Remedy

The remedy softens the personality and leads them to look within for the qualities needed to accomplish their tasks in life. They learn how to lead people rather than drive them. They find the wisdom to use a softer, more balanced approach to achieve their ends. It is not so much that they are wrong in what they try to achieve, after all the world needs decisive strong leaders, but the remedy helps them to contact their inner intuitive leadership ability, rather than working from a state of arrogance.

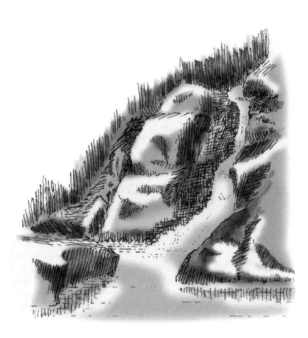

Qualities of Rock Water

The persistent but gentle action of water can change the shape and attitude of a rock face. The apparently weaker water shapes and smoothes the jagged edges of seemingly impervious rock. The interaction between the rock face and the water shows us how overly rigid ideals can be changed by persistent gentle persuasion rather than by aggressive force. Rock water also carries healing energy from the depths of the earth helping to connect us to the wisdom of the planet.

Chakra Qualities

Brow – *6th Chakra*
Rainbow Colour – Indigo

This is the quality of change, the ability to take new ideas and allow life to flow on and situations to change. We are free from the need of rigid form in our lives to enable us to feel safe.

Positive Qualities

We have the unique quality of empathy combined with flexibility of mind and purpose. We develop a strong connection to the ever-changing world and are tolerant if not positive about change. By allowing ourselves to go with the flow we follow our natural path and by flowing with the changes that are necessary we ensure that we remain connected to our source.

Negative State

Rock water essence is helpful if we have found a philosophy or approach to life that we hold to be absolutely true. We may not try to convert others to our viewpoint but we are unable to see that we could bend in any way concerning our own views. We have placed the whole of our faith in an external view of life, placing no trust whatever in our own inner guidance. We totally ignore that still small voice within that could lead us to the truth.

The Action of the Remedy

Rock water is not a flower remedy. It is water taken from a healing spring. When Dr. Bach was looking for a remedy for this very rigid type of personality he noticed that spring water would even wear away something as hard and rigid as a rock, so in time it will even wear down and soften a rigid personality. When the personality has softened it is able to look within for guidance rather than without to rigid form and structure.

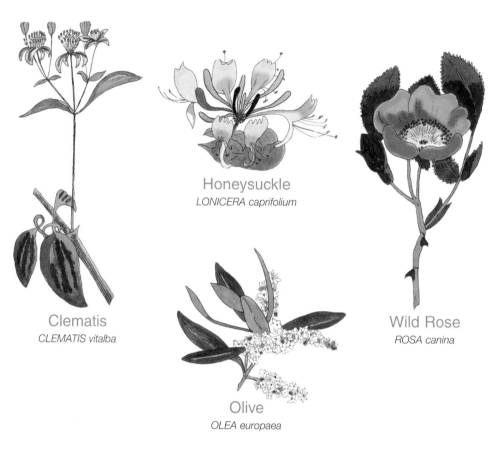

Clematis
CLEMATIS vitalba

Honeysuckle
LONICERA caprifolium

Wild Rose
ROSA canina

Olive
OLEA europaea

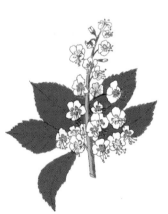

White Chestnut
AESCULUS hippocastanum

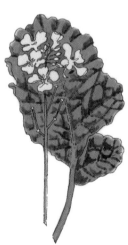

Mustard
SINAPSIS arvensis

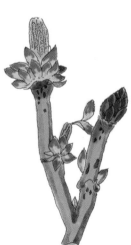

Chestnut Bud
AESCULUS hippocastanum

CHAPTER 7

Throat Chakra and Remedies
Rainbow Colour Blue

Energy Quality – Ether
5th Age – From 28 Years to 35 Years

The energetic expressions of this Chakra are space, as the perfect form of all things, and time, as the unfolding of the divine plan at its rightful pace and place in creation.

Our blueprint, which holds the plan or pattern for our life and health is held at this etheric level and all experiences at all levels affect this Chakra. It enables us to communicate, change, and heal at all levels. The Throat Chakra is the connecting Chakra between the lower spiritual and higher mind energies. Spirit is without form, and mind is the realm of form. This Chakra is referred to as the mind or causal level of creation. When out of balance, we disconnect from being in the 'here and now': we lose our plan, repeat negative patterns, display a tendency to avoid the present by dreamy absent mindedness and a lack of concentration, living in the past, brooding on the future, going over and over things in the mind in an attempt 'to get it right' rather than resting on divine wisdom and love. We find difficulty in communicating and are unable to allow our own healing or readjusting to take place, which would in turn reconnect us with our divine plan. Eventually, this disconnectedness can lead to complete mental and emotional exhaustion, and possibly breakdown.

Remedy Group
Lack of interest in present circumstances

Remedies
Clematis, Honeysuckle, Wild Rose, Olive, White Chestnut,
Mustard, Chestnut Bud

The Flower

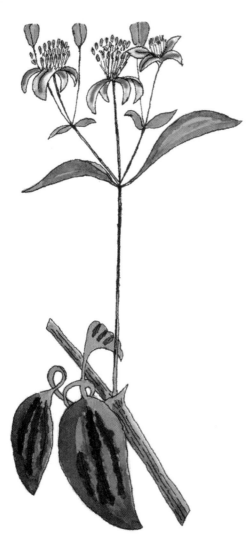

Qualities of the Flower

Clematis reaches for the sky with its beautiful flowers. However the plant can seem to live in its top airy-fairy flowers with the woody stem seeming barren with no live connection between the flowers and the roots.

Chakra Qualities

Throat – *5th Chakra*
Rainbow Colour – Blue

To be able to bring to the plan or vision of the Throat Chakra into the physical or to current reality we must be in a state of groundedness. If we are not grounded, our ideas, visions and aspirations will remain as such and will not be brought into physical reality. The action of this Chakra is healing and communication.

Positive Qualities

This is the energy of being grounded yet with a lively interest in life. Having a clear vision of where we are going and how we are going to get there. This gives us a relaxed approach to life, which is completely focused and positive. We are also capable of inspiring others, helping to build the vision of a better future.

Negative State

Clematis is indicated when a person is dreamy and disconnected from reality. They are vague and unfocused, wandering around in a mental fog. Their lives are always in a mess because they can never concentrate sufficiently to complete the task in hand. The many things which are left uncompleted and still demanding attention, just add to general chaos. Their desires always seem unattainable or out of reach. They seem incapable of materialising their desires and dreams. They live for the future when things will be better.

The Action of the Remedy

The remedy opens the gate between the mind and physical reality. It brings the energy to a point where aspirations and dreams can crystallize and come into being in the physical world.

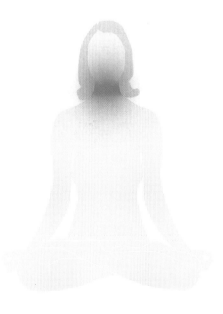

Flower

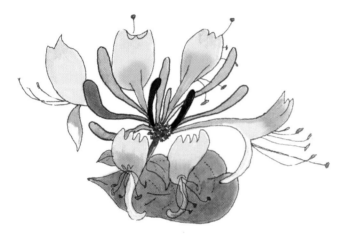

Qualities of the Flower

Honeysuckle is prolific in its growth producing an abundance of flowers but if allowed to become too overgrown it creates a tangled mess from which it can barely move. It is instantly recognisable by its strong sweet scent. If it does not have a clear space to grow in, it can become matted and dense with what appears to be masses of dead wood.

Chakra Qualities

Throat – *5th Chakra*
Rainbow Colour – Blue

We are connected to our true vibration through our blueprint at the Throat level. This quality is about being in the now. To realise our potential we must be able to live in our present.

Positive Qualities

We have the ability to retain the wisdom gained from past experiences without wallowing in nostalgia. When we let go of the past, we can love it or loathe it without being stuck in it. This allows us to focus on the task in hand and look forward to the future with confidence.

Negative State

In this state people live in the past. They escape current reality by harking back to some supposedly idyllic time when everything was better, or bitterly regretting the hard times when there were no opportunities, or when circumstances stopped them making the most of themselves. Their lives lack focus because either it can never be as good now as it was then so they have no positive future focus, or as the opportunities were lost in the past, they can only see a repetition of the same pattern. If we are constantly reliving the past we are unable to move forward or to bring our future into the present. The feeling is 'My time has past!'

The Action of the Remedy

The remedy helps to clear the illusion of an over idyllic past or helps to release the need to repeat the pattern of past trauma. When the past is accepted and released, it is then possible for our attention to be on the task in hand. People find it easy to resolve life's challenges once they can focus on them and deal with them. The remedy helps us to live in and deal with the NOW.

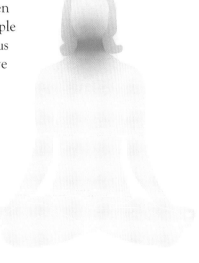

The Flower

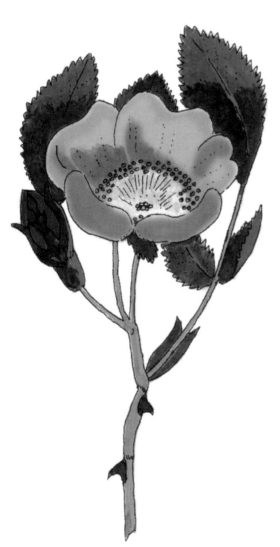

Qualities of the Flower

The wild rose is the crowning glory that adds beauty and serenity to many hedgerows. It has been one of the symbols of the British Monarchy since the 1500s. It has been used for many years as a source of vitamin C, obtained from its lush red fruit in the form of rosehip syrup.

Chakra Qualities

Throat – *5th Chakra*
Rainbow Colour – Blue

This Chakra gives us the connection we need to realise our full potential and to BE fully in our lives rather than simply doing things in them. Our path may not always appear easy and we need a strong connection to our vision to be able to maintain our focus without being overwhelmed.

Positive Qualities

These are people who are excited and enthusiastic about life. They grasp the power and joy of the moment when any task presents itself to them and set about it with vigour. They love to be the centre of attention and live in the swim of life.

Negative State

Wild rose is needed when anyone feels like giving up on life. The struggle is too much. Disconnected from life and resigned to whatever happens, in this state things just drift along. The person is overwhelmed because they do not have a true sense of their full potential. They are unable to heal because the energy that would enable healing has been disconnected from within. Their vision dissolves in the onslaught of what seems to be nothing but insurmountable problems.

The Action of the Remedy

The remedy helps to reconnect us to the energy of our intended path in life, at the Throat Chakra. Once the connection is made we can then perceive the perfect form of our full potential, allowing us to heal and realise every facet of our individuality. We see a vision of how wonderful our life really is and enthusiastically plunge back into the joy of being.

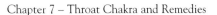

The Flower

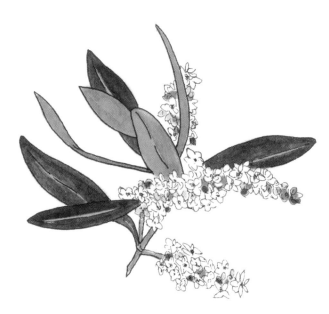

Qualities of the Flower

The long-term commitment of the man who plants an olive tree for the benefit of future generations, reflects the quality of the olive tree. It demands patience and persistence and a faith that the end product will be worth the wait. Once it begins to bear fruit its yield increases each year until maturity. It can continue to fruit for hundreds of years.

Chakra Qualities

Throat – *5th Chakra*
Rainbow Colour – Blue

To be able to create our reality we must hold our vision until it is realised. Through whatever trials and difficulties that beset us we need to maintain the balance at all levels and a connection to the lower physical qualities while waiting for the vision to manifest and then holding onto that vision to continue the process over the years.

Positive Qualities

The persistence to hold a long-term vision without giving up on it before it is achieved. This is the type of person who with great strength of mind works with a calm resolute focus on the vision. They have the ability to see a task through to completion whatever obstacles may arise or however long it takes. Positive olive people keep going when the going gets tough and others are falling by the wayside. They are then able to continue to hold the vision and build on their success year on year for as long as the vision is viable.

Negative State

Olive is often prescribed for exhaustion but this is not the exhaustion of fatigue caused by overwork, but the exhaustion that comes when the mind can take no more and snaps. It is the exhaustion of the person who gives up when the goal is in sight and victory might be won with just a little more effort. The mind gives up and the will is sapped as the tightly held focus on the vision is lost.

The Action of the Remedy

This remedy helps the person who faces enormous challenges in life to hold on to their vision. It helps to hold the focus while waiting for things to manifest and then to keep the flow of manifestation going. It connects us with the inner strength needed to continue this focus on the vision and regain physical strength to carry on, without fear that their resolve will be lost.

The Tree

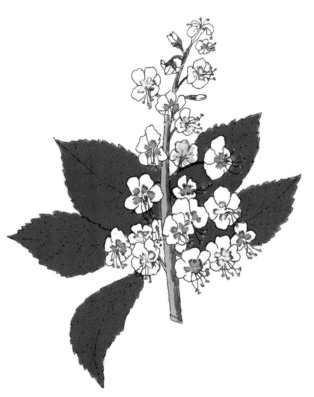

Qualities of the Tree

Made up of delicate small white flowers, the candle like groups of the white chestnut blossom portrays intense detail. The overall beauty of this majestic tree exudes a sense of peace and harmony. It is the mature version of chestnut bud.

Chakra Qualities

Throat – *5th Chakra*
Rainbow Colour – Blue

It is the quality of clarity of vision without confusion or turmoil. It is the sense of being in the now in our own power.

Positive Qualities

When we can work on a problem with a calm clear mind unaffected by outside influences, we have the ability to sort out the mess when a situation has gone out of control. When faced with any situation, we quietly set about deciding exactly what needs to be done. Then we can resolve the problem in a clear untroubled way. We have a clear view of the target and the focus to put all of our energy behind 'our arrow', which makes hitting the target much easier.

Negative State

The negative white chestnut can never get a clear vision of the solution to a problem. Working at it first from this point of view and then from that point of view, people go over the whole situation again and again without rest or resolution. They exhaust themselves with too much thinking and still never get to the point where a solution can be found.

The Action of the Remedy

The remedy helps us to cut through the dross of our own confusing mental processes. We then get a clear view of the resolution we are searching for. The energy that previously was used in useless mental turmoil can now be used to solve the problem.

The Flower

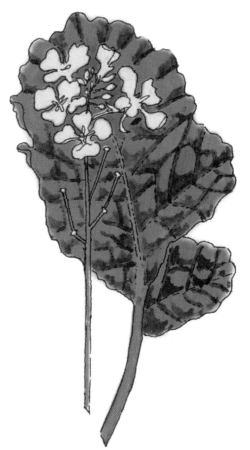

Qualities of the Flower

This light yellow flower has the ability to wait for the right conditions for its germination and will grow after long periods of time being inactive. It seems to appear 'out of the blue'.

Chakra Qualities

Throat – *5th Chakra*
Rainbow Colour – Blue

This quality is of having faith to not lose our confidence when we know our goal, but are suddenly disorientated around it. When we are certain of our goal we feel safe. Even if it is not manifesting immediately, we are prepared to bide our time until conditions are right.

Positive Qualities

This remedy gives us an unshakeable inner serenity and connection to the present. It connects us to a state of constant stability and joy.

Negative State

This is indicated by depression that comes out of a clear blue sky, for no apparent reason. Nothing helps to lift it; friends who try just make things worse. It can seem that all hope is lost. Then, just as quickly and for no apparent reason, the depression lifts, the sun comes out and all is well with the world. For some deep psychological reason the person who suffers from this condition loses their vision of the ideal at the Throat Chakra, and with it goes their natural sense that things will work out: hence the sudden sense of abject despondency and the typifying and immediate depression.

The Action of the Remedy

The remedy helps the sufferer to locate and face the condition that is causing the problem. It is only by finding and facing our demons that we can clear them. Taking the remedy can in some cases lead to a period of additional trauma as the inner blocks are faced and dealt with. When this happens successfully, then the demons can be laid to rest for good, the vision is clearly held and a sense of trust pervades lifting the depression.

The Tree

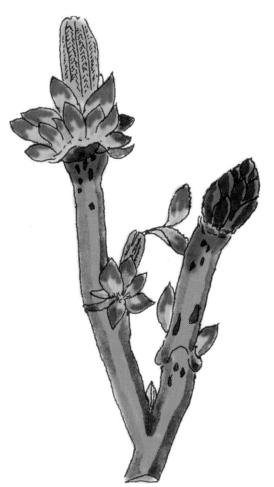

Qualities of the Tree

The state prior to flowering is when the bud is at its most vulnerable and must trust its true potential before moving forward to a more glorious state. This is the bud state of the white chestnut.

Chakra Qualities

Throat – *5th Chakra*
Rainbow Colour – Blue

This quality is about taking information and lessons we need to learn so as to clear distortions at the Throat Chakra level (i.e. in the blueprint), in order to allow unhindered progress along our true-life path.

Positive Qualities

With this quality we are keen observers of life and learn from our experiences. It is about attention to the now and what is necessary to move on without repeating the mistakes of the past. We are able to move forward using past experiences to develop our potential. We find it easy to absorb and assimilate information and are good students.

Negative State

In this state people never learn from their mistakes. They repeat the same drama or get into the same mess time and time again. Everyone around them is at a loss to understand how they can be 'in that situation again'. This can also be seen in students who are clearly competent but the lessons somehow are not remembered. They forget everything they were taught as they walk out of the classroom at the end of the lecture.

The Action of the Remedy

The remedy helps these people to contact the energy of the Throat Chakra. This will enable them to release the distortion that blocks understanding. This will allow them to understand at a deep level of their being what it is they are expected to learn. This then makes it possible to learn and thereby develop, grow and move on to new lessons in life.

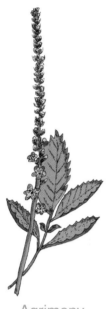

Agrimony

AGRIMONIA eupatoria

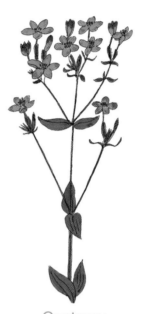

Centaury

ERYTHRAEA centaurium

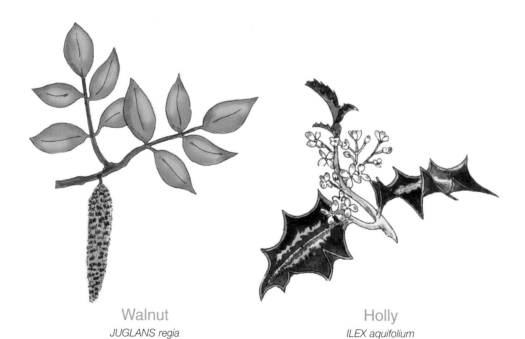

Walnut

JUGLANS regia

Holly

ILEX aquifolium

CHAPTER 8

Heart Chakra and Remedies

Rainbow Colour Green

Energy Quality – Air
4th Age – From 21 Years to 28 Years

This Chakra is associated with love and compassion, and as love has the capacity to change anything and anybody, so this centre transforms the incoming mental / spiritual energies into the more tangible lower mind energies of our physical world. Likewise the returning physical energies transmute through the heart centre to return to the higher mind and spiritual consciousness.

This process engenders heartfelt love for all, dedication and self-realisation, to connect us with our true desire, warmth, spontaneity, and openness. Imbalance expresses itself in a lack of confidence in our own desires, dreams, plans, and judgement. This manifests as self-doubt, suspicion, anger, and a feeling of struggle between body and mind.

Remedy Group
Over sensitivity to influences and ideas

Remedies
Agrimony, Centaury, Walnut, Holly

The Flower

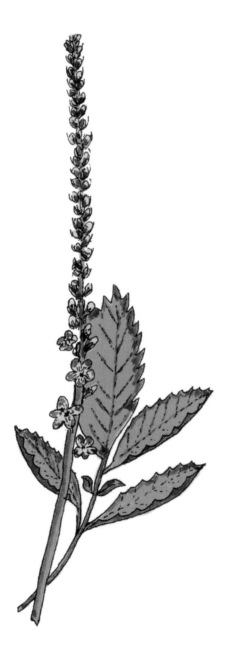

Qualities of the Flower

The very pretty cluster of small yellow flowers make up what seem like fingers pointing skywards. They seem intent on a goal, displaying a strong self-reliance and individuality.

Chakra Qualities

Heart – *4th Chakra*
Rainbow Colour – Green

The ability to be strong through adversity, whilst responding appropriately to stress and difficulties. A balanced heart has the quality of flexibility with strength.

Positive Qualities

To be truly resilient, not hiding behind a false front of smiles. These people are life's optimists. They have a genuine personality, which is both engaging and embracing. They exude heartfelt warmth and humour, and have strength of heart, which is fearless in adversity: they are true heroes.

Negative State

Those in agrimony's negative state are very sensitive, and will go to great lengths to avoid quarrels or disharmony. This sensitivity may cause nervous restlessness but they will make light of the situation or condition and may even joke about it rather than admit there is a problem or accept help. They may even resort to alcohol or drugs to quieten the inner pain. They will maintain an outer show of confidence, with a brave face and assurances that they are 'fine', whilst experiencing inner turmoil.

The Action of the Remedy

The remedy helps to calm and focus the energy of the Heart Chakra so that the sufferer can achieve a true inner calm and balance. The problem may arise from a heart that is too open and therefore feels vulnerable. They are keen to know what is happening but are not confident enough in their desire to trust their judgement or to fight for their beliefs. The suffering is released when the open heart can trust its judgement and feel truly cheerful, jovial and happy, from the heart without the need to 'put on a brave face'.

The Flower

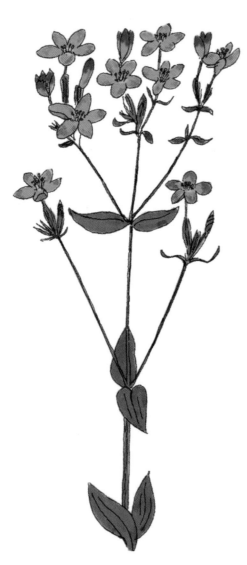

Qualities of the Flower

This plant can be easily missed while you are out walking. Like a centurion at the gate, it does nothing to attract attention. It has confidence in its own right to be here in the world and it is content not to be the centre of attention. If you take the time to look carefully, you will appreciate the strength in the beautifully delicate pink flowers.

Chakra Qualities

Heart – *4th Chakra*
Rainbow Colour – Green

The quality is that of allowing the heart its full potential to love, including ourselves. We are not able to truly love another until we love and accept ourselves: not as a perfect being but with all our imperfections. This plant is said to be named after the centaur Chiron, known in Astrological circles as the wounded healer. He used the plant to cure himself of a wound inflicted by the nine-headed serpent Hydra.

Positive Qualities

A strong character, knowing when to give, and when to be firm. One who can offer true service to others because they are never servile. They serve from the heart, from the pure joy and pleasure of offering service to another person.

Negative State

Negative centaury people are in a weak-willed state which is eager to please, to the point where they will often become a drudge simply because they never complain. They just drift into the most menial tasks. These are often people whose heart has been most grievously wounded, so much so that they will do anything to please rather than risk the pain which may come from standing up to others even when they know that they are being taken advantage of. The heart is so weak they are often pale from the inability of the heart to pump blood around the body. It feels as though there is not enough to go round. In trying to serve everyone else's needs, they omit to address their own.

The Action of the Remedy

The remedy helps to release the pain and heal the heart so that the sufferer can once again face the world with a brave heart. They can then stand up for themselves from true inner strength without being put upon. They achieve the strength to become balanced and once again easily transmute the positive heart energies. Once their wounds are healed they are then in a position to be of service and to impart strength to all those who need succour, empowering others to help themselves.

Flower

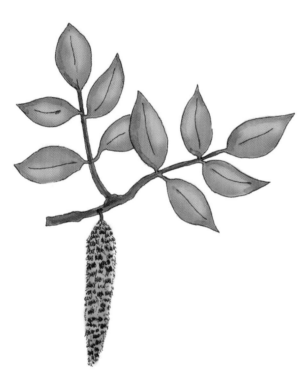

Qualities of the Flower

The Greeks called the walnut the 'royal' nut or 'persian' nut, names which reflect its importance and its origin. The fruit of the walnut resembles the brain. The walnut shell protects the fruit while allowing it to grow and develop just as the bones of the cranium protect the brain without inhibiting energy flowing through it.

Chakra Qualities

Heart – *4th Chakra*
Rainbow Colour – Green

The heart is the meeting point of spiritual energy descending into physicality and physical energy ascending into a spiritual state. This quality brings with it the ability to move on through the transitions we must experience as part of our life's path.

Positive Qualities

Walnut gives us the wonderful quality of strength with balance. We have the strength and subtlety to handle changing circumstances without being thrown off course. We feel safe and within our boundaries, even though those boundaries are changing or expanding.

Negative State

We are rendered vulnerable by life's circumstances, unable to move on without feeling broken and damaged by the changes in our life. Walnut is recommended when people undergo major changes in life, to the extent that the very foundations of life feel threatened. This can happen at times when the changes are natural and expected such as the birth of a child, puberty, the teenage years, or menopause, as well as the changes that life thrusts on us such as redundancy or bankruptcy, career change, the breakdown of a relationship, divorce, children leaving home, moving house or country. At these times there is a massive increase in the flow of energy through the heart to deal with the new situation. This increased energy flow is more obvious during puberty or menopause when not only mental energies, but physical energies are vastly increased to deal with the changes. During these changes, even a balanced heart can be destabilized by the increased flow of energy. Walnut is also indicated when the problems are dealt with by disconnecting from the flow and becoming hard hearted.

The Action of the Remedy

The remedy helps us to find the strength to deal with changing situations without losing balance. This does not mean that we will not experience some of the pain of change. This is inevitable at times of high drama, but with the help of the remedy we are able to cope and retain our connection with our self and our path and maintain a sense of our place and our right to be. We are supported in the balance of physical and spiritual flow.

Flower

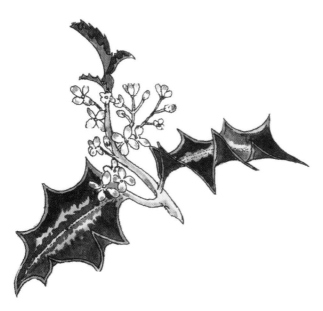

Qualities of the Flower

The holly once established is a very robust, resilient shrub. Its leaves make it a superb 'protector'. There was a belief that it was unlucky to cut down a holly tree, and it has long been associated with eternity and thought to ward off evil and destruction. It grows in most soils, and is a vibrant presence in all seasons even bearing its gift of vibrant red berries to us at Christmas. It is however not to be tangled with, as its spiked leaves are very sharp.

Chakra Qualities

Heart – *4th Chakra*
Rainbow Colour – Green

This quality of the Heart Chakra is about unconditional love – not closed or holding on to past hurt. This is the quality of understanding that every incarnate soul on this planet is created from the energy of pure love. When we express this energy we have the capacity to draw universal love through ourselves and send powerful waves of it into everything and everybody around us.

Positive Qualities

These people are warm-hearted, loving and generous. They radiate love and happiness to all and are tolerant of the failings and shortcomings of others.

Negative State

Holly in this state is the opposite of heartfelt love, displaying emotions such as jealousy, bitterness, anger, envy, suspicion, rage, selfishness or any emotion which cuts off the heart energies of joy, openness and love for all. The heart energies become distorted and bitter, the body becomes gnarled and withered as the positive energies, which bring elegance and poise, no longer flow through the heart.

The Action of the Remedy

The remedy soothes and softens the over protectiveness of the heart to enable the more positive energies to flow once again releasing the negative emotions harboured within the heart. This manifests as a brightening and softening of the features: friends say we look years younger. We feel as though a great burden has been lifted from our shoulders as heartfelt emotions become more positive, suddenly there is a spring in our steps and we are open hearted and joyous once again. Along with crab apple, which cleans the aura, this remedy is ideal for therapists to ensure they do not 'pick up' negative energy from their clients.

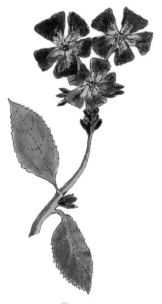

Cerato

CERATOSTIGMA willmottiana

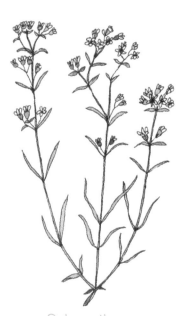

Scleranthus

SCLERANTHUS annus

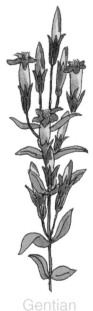

Gentian

GENTIANA amarella

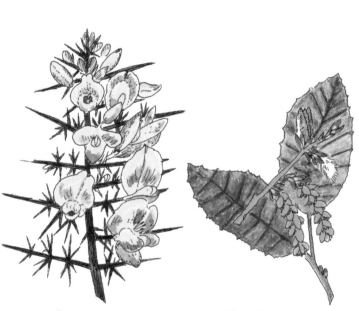

Gorse

UKX europaeus

Hornbeam

CARPINUS betulus

Wild Oat

BROMUS asper

CHAPTER 9

Solar Plexus Chakra
and Remedies
Rainbow Colour Yellow

Energy Quality – Fire
3rd Age – From 14 Years to 21 Years

Often referred to as the brain of the body, this is the centre from which all automatic and learned functions emanate, and it houses our ability to do and be as an individual in the world. Logical thinking and feeling are central to this Chakra. At this level, the energy demands certainty, and is unbalanced by a lack of direction and understanding. The higher spiritual energies guide us into right action, seeing the wider and further vision. Once a line of action is decided, the Solar Plexus Chakra is happy and will function to fuel the transformation of desire or plans into physical reality.

An imbalance leads us to be out of harmony with our driving force, unable to see our right path or trust that it is there. We lack direction becoming apathetic and indecisive which leads to fear and anxiety.

Remedy Group
Uncertainty

Remedies
Cerato, Scleranthus, Gentian, Gorse, Hornbeam, Wild Oat

Flower

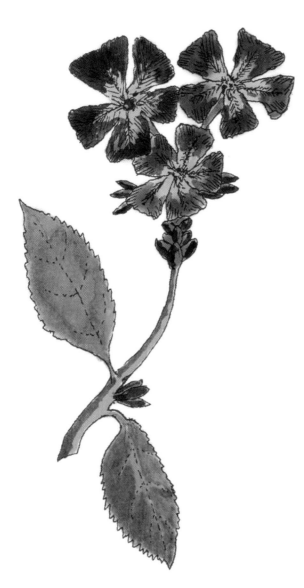

Qualities of the Flower

The flower is a vividly intense violet blue with five wedge shaped petals. It originated on the Tibetan border of China and was bought to England in 1908. It is found in gardens where it is cultivated as an ornamental shrub.

Chakra Qualities

Solar Plexus – *3rd Chakra*
Rainbow Colour – Yellow

This is the quality of certainty in all we think, say and do. It is our connection through the Throat Chakra to the Brow and Crown Chakras – our thirst for our own inner truth.

Positive Qualities

We have the ability to take direct and correct action on intuitive impulse. Everybody in the world acts, but the ability to 'see' what the need is in any situation and take decisive action to bring about a beneficial outcome, is a unique ability.

Negative State

In a negative cerato state, people cannot make a decision. It isn't that they don't have enough facts or information: it is that the information goes continually around in their head so they cannot decide. They lack inner conviction, no matter how many facts or how much information is put before them. They simply 'do not have the guts' to make the decision. They could ask twenty people for their advice, yet even if they got the same information from everyone, they still would not have the guts to decide. They have such a deep anxiety, it deprives them of the courage to make a decision.

The Action of the Remedy

The remedy helps them to release the anxiety, thereby enabling them to act on the vision from the Brow and Throat Chakras with the necessary courage to take action. They are reconnected with their inner counsel and are no longer too fearful to act. The strength of certainty at the Solar Plexus is restored and confidence in their own ability is re-established.

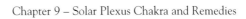

Flower

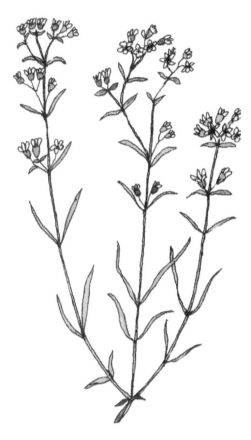

Qualities of the Flower

This plant likes dry sandy or gravely places to grow. It is small and has a wiry, bushy appearance. Dividing into many stems just above the root, it has narrow pointed leaves and green flowers with no petals that are less than 4mm across. The stems of this plant suggest dealing with a constant changing of direction. It has no difficulty deciding which way to grow: it simply grows in as many directions as it wishes to.

Chakra Qualities

Solar Plexus – *3rd Chakra*
Rainbow Colour – Yellow

The quality is of steadfast focus on our goals and outcomes – this where we set our life aims and goals. It is the energy of structure: as the energy of the Heart Chakra (desire) moves down, the action required to achieve the desire is decided.

Positive Qualities

This is demonstrated in a person who is well balanced, instinctively knowing what action to take, they trust their intuition and act resolutely on their intuitive impulse. This is the quality of true decisiveness, not panic decision-making.

Negative State

In a negative scleranthus state, people are simply unable to make up their minds. They have the courage to make a decision, but they may change the decision twenty times in as many minutes. Their energy vacillates between this and that, without coming to one decision, and sticking to it. It is an inner state of confusion, which is very difficult to pin down. In fact they do not even know whether they need a remedy or not.

The Action of the Remedy

The remedy enables them to gain inner balance and composure, which gives them the focus to make a decision, stick with it, and act. It strengthens the connection to both the Heart and Sacral Chakras so we are able to identify our desire and so the fire of the Solar Plexus Chakra can be used by the Sacral Chakra to create the outcome we want. The will is strengthened, and it transforms the anxiety or fear of making a wrong decision. Interestingly this remedy is very good for seasickness, which is a moving around between this and that. The remedy itself will bring about sufficient healing to achieve a state of balance. Remember the remedy itself will not ensure that a correct decision will be made. For that we still need connection to the higher Chakras to connect us to the fountain of wisdom.

Flower

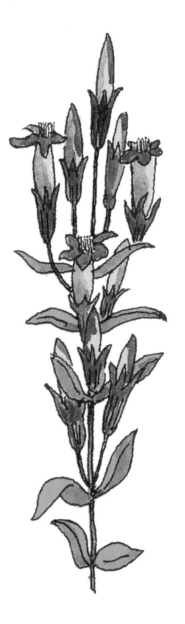

Qualities of the Flower

This plant is a late flowerer. It has the patience to wait all summer long until its flowers are ready to express their full potential. It prefers high hillside or hill top spots as if it is trying to reach out to the sky. It is a tall plant with strong upright purple, blue or violet trumpet-like flowers.

Chakra Qualities

Solar Plexus – *3rd Chakra*
Rainbow Colour – Yellow

This quality gives the Solar Plexus Chakra its constancy of connection with the higher Chakras, keeping us in touch with a greater understanding of our purpose, and connected with the abundant vital energy needed to keep going.

Positive Qualities

This is reflected in people who have the resolve to see a task through to completion. They see what needs to be done, brush aside setbacks and get on with the job in hand. Their clarity and focus enables them to face adversity courageously and act to bring about the desired outcome resolutely.

Negative State

In a negative gentian state we see people getting along fine when suddenly there is a minor set back. They immediately become depressed and feel that their efforts will end in failure. They are the natural sceptics of the world, almost taking refuge in melancholy. They 'knew it would not work out anyway' and can always tell you the reason why. The depression is always out of proportion to the challenge faced. They wallow in a pervasive gloom, which breeds a sense of failure.

The Action of the Remedy

The remedy can lift the fog, which blocks out the sun of their Solar Plexus Chakra. The reason for their melancholy is that they have lost contact with the higher energies, which would give them the faith to enable them to meet and overcome their difficulties. The remedy helps them to reconnect to their ability to trust that anything is possible if they believe in it enough. The connection to their source enables the trust that although things appear to be stuck or failing, a process is being played out. They cease to buy into failure and create success through divine intention and trust that everything will work to their greater good.

Flower

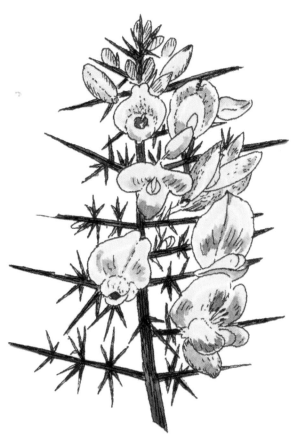

Qualities of the Flower

Gorse has very bright yellow flowers that brighten the landscape from spring until late summer and sometimes into the winter, bringing a sense of sunshine in all weathers. It is protected by huge spiky leaves and has amazing resilience. There is an old saying that while gorse flowers in an area, it will never be conquered.

Chakra Qualities

Solar Plexus – *3rd Chakra*
Rainbow Colour – Yellow

This quality of the Solar Plexus Chakra is our connection to vibrant life. It is our get up and go, to tackle any challenge and move forward.

Positive Qualities

We demonstrate a positive gorse state when we radiate joy and vitality. We hold an inner conviction that the outcome to any endeavour will be positive. We have a natural and unassuming faith in our ability to succeed and have the drive and stamina to keep going until we achieve what we desire. A robust person with a fiery Solar Plexus Chakra would deal with problems that defeat a negative gorse type, with little effort or concern in the normal course of getting on with their day.

Negative State

In a negative gorse state, people have a sallow complexion and an air of deep resignation and despair. The sun of their Solar Plexus Chakra is not just blocked by fog: it has all but gone out, there is no fuel to drive the system to enable it to overcome its negativity. The lack of fire shows in the sallow complexion. These people do not have enough 'fire in the belly' to face what the world throws at them and deal with it. They have 'lost heart'.

The Action of the Remedy

The bright yellow flowers of gorse help to feed the furnace of the Solar Plexus Chakra with the energy it needs to lift the sufferer to the point where they can throw off the melancholy. This enables them to face the world with enough 'fire in the belly' to easily face and deal with the problems which life throws up. The remedy reconnects the fire of the Solar Plexus Chakra to the desire of the heart, helping to lighten the heart and so raise their expectations. This allows the light into their lives again. Interestingly, the herbs that stimulate the fire energy are nearly all bitter. So when you taste a bitter herb, you are stimulating the fire energy to help you throw off the disease.

Tree

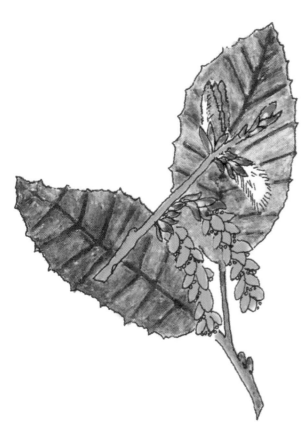

Qualities of the Tree

This tree is of exceptionally strong wood. The name 'horn' gives an idea of its strength. (Beam being the old name for tree). It has many uses thanks to its solid strength. It used to be coppiced or pollarded and has long been used for hedgerows, growing so thickly and holding onto many dead leaves in winter that gives some privacy all the year round.

Chakra Qualities

Solar Plexus – *3rd Chakra*
Rainbow Colour – Yellow

The Solar Plexus Chakra provides the fire energy that is used to enliven, animate and drive the other energies in the body. Without the fire of the Solar Plexus Chakra, the other energies would be dormant and inactive.

Positive Qualities

The positive hornbeam quality is that of vibrant energy easily focused on the task in hand. They have a bright joyous outlook: a person whose inner strength leads them to seek out and enjoy challenges. They have lots of get up and go.

Negative State

The negative hornbeam feeling is simply a state of low fire energy. We would recognise it as the Monday morning feeling, where someone just needs some encouragement and a little push to get them going. If you have ever noticed your energy dropping after you have been working for a long time, try this experiment. Take a break and some hornbeam and in a few minutes you will feel refreshed and creative, much more so than if you had just had a break without any hornbeam.

The Action of the Remedy

This remedy simply gives a little boost to the fire energy of the Solar Plexus Chakra, to get it going. It strengthens the connection to the red energy of the Base Chakra. This is not a remedy for deep mental or physical exhaustion, but one that helps us to deal with the mundane affairs of life with less difficulty. Rather like a brisk walk that enlivens and animates us to enable us to tackle the tasks at hand with ease.

Flower

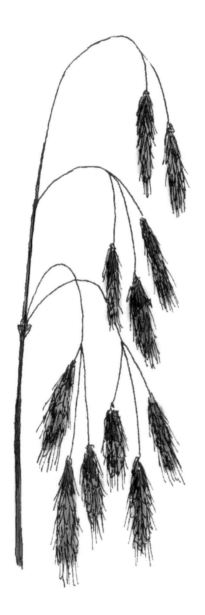

Qualities of the Flower

The seeds of the wild oat seem to 'hang about' waiting for some divine force to decide where they should go and what they should do. Of course each seed has its destined direction, usually a hedgerow, and it grows and thrives seemingly without struggle.

Chakra Qualities

Solar Plexus – *3rd Chakra*
Rainbow Colour – Yellow

This strand of Solar Plexus energy is focused on the Brow Chakra. It is about our ability to see the big picture, to bring in the vision, seeing it with certainty and direction.

Positive Qualities

The positive wild oat person has a clear vision of the future, who can 'see' the outcome they wish to achieve. They are ambitious and know what action to take when faced with a challenge. They recognise their path in life and follow it until the outcome they have envisioned is achieved.

Negative State

In a negative wild oat state people have lost the greater vision. They cannot make progress because they are lost in the minutiae of life. Let's face it: nobody is stimulated to make Herculean effort in life just to get a lousy job to pay the rent. We are all born with a mission in life. This is not necessarily something that will place us in the public eye or make us materially rich, but it is one that will bring great satisfaction and sufficient material rewards to live abundantly within our chosen lifestyle. The remedy is useful when we need to see our way forward in life, when choosing a career or making a lifestyle change. This is sometimes referred to as following our pathway or song line through life. If you are bored with your life, this is a good indication that you are not on your song line and need to take wild oat.

The Action of the Remedy

This remedy re-connects us to our Brow Chakra, which in turn enables us to clear our vision and use the insight that is now available to us, to see the way ahead. The Solar Plexus Chakra can get on with the germination of ideas, giving shape to the plans we have for our life. This can be illustrated by the way a seed holds the vision that the plant grows into. Another way to look at this is that as the mist clears, we are able to see the snow capped mountains in the distance which are our goal.

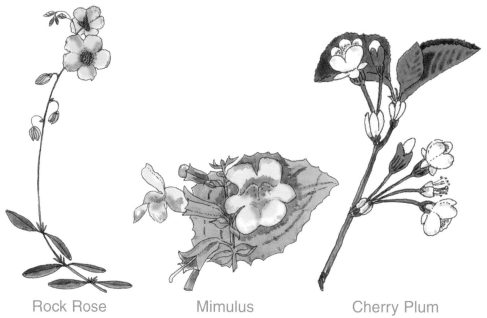

Rock Rose

HELIANTHEMUM vulgare

Mimulus

MIMULUS luteus

Cherry Plum

PRUNUS cerasifera

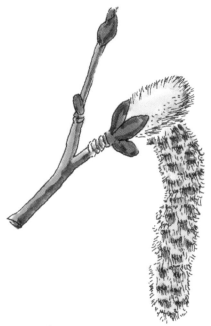

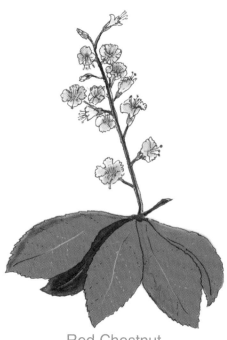

Aspen

POPULUS tremula

Red Chestnut

AESCULUS carnea

CHAPTER 10

Sacral Chakra and Remedies
Rainbow Colour Orange

Energy Quality – Water
2nd Age – From 7 Years to 14 Years

This is the centre of physical creation, the procreation of the human race. From the expression of an art form into physical reality, or of an idea jotted on a scrap of paper seen through to a successful business. The emotional input needed to create at this level requires the ability to be able to relate to others with trust and openness, able to share, trade and exchange with them for mutual benefit.

Vitality, creativity, emotional sexuality, and anything experienced as a flowing wave-like watery movement are the key energies of this Chakra.

Shock or trauma held at this level will affect our relationships in all aspects of our lives. We become fearful or even panic stricken. This brings about a rigidity which blocks our ability to relate to others in a positive and meaningful way. The potential for successful partnerships can be impaired until the underlying imbalance is faced and cleared.

Remedy Group
Fear

Remedies
Rock Rose, Mimulus, Cherry Plum, Aspen, Red Chestnut

Flower

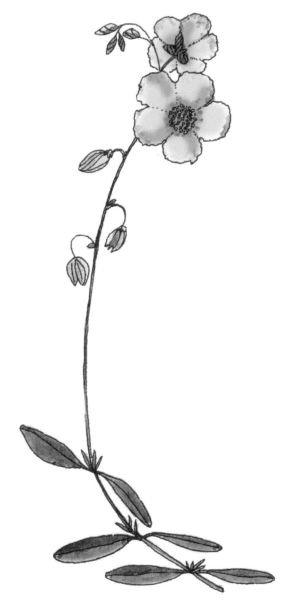

Qualities of the Flower

This is a very delicate looking plant. Growing in somewhat inhospitable areas, it seems happy to grow in not much more than shale or shingle (rocks) or chalk. It has bright flowers and can grow anywhere, bringing colour to otherwise desolate places.

Chakra Qualities

Sacral – *2nd Chakra*
Rainbow Colour – Orange

Moving with the flow of life. Dealing with everything with confidence, poise and balance.

Positive Qualities

This is the courage to take action once the decision has been made, and to have a clear conviction of a positive outcome of one's actions. This conviction brings bravery or even heroism in the face of adversity.

Negative State

In a negative rock rose state, people are prone to becoming fearful, panic stricken and rigid with fear when faced with an emergency. Because the emotional centre is disturbed, they can be subject to night terrors, nightmares, or horrors of unknown origin. This state is the exact opposite of the beautiful emotions of emotional love. Emotional imbalances cause the sufferer to lose contact with the positive qualities of the Sacral Chakra. All that is felt and exhibited are the dramatic, negative, fearful qualities.

The Action of the Remedy

The remedy brings warmth back to this centre from the fire of the Solar Plexus Chakra and it creates the calming soothing warmth of a big beautiful orange sunset on a warm summer evening. As the vibrations at this centre lift, life becomes calmer, the dark storm of emotion passes, and the person becomes much more receptive to help.

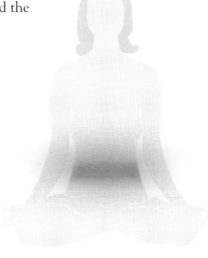

Flower

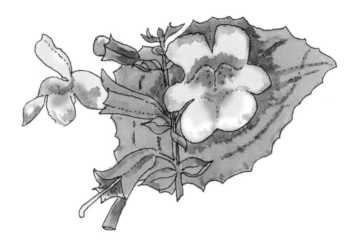

Qualities of the Flower

These vibrant plants flower freely at the side of rivers and streams with no apparent thought for their own safety. Their yellow flowers are speckled with red, which seems to reflect the very essence of the life giving sun.

Chakra Qualities

Sacral – *2nd Chakra*
Rainbow Colour – Orange

This ebb and flow energy quality connects our Base Chakra through the Sacral Chakra to higher aspirations than material gain. It holds the trust that we have all things necessary to feel secure.

Positive Qualities

These are people who have a clear, unworried mind. It is not that they do not face challenges in life, but that they have a balanced serenity. They have a quality of gentle courage, which allows them to enjoy life to the full.

Negative State

Mimulus is indicated when the fear is known. It may or may not be logical. When we stand back from life through fear, it may be fear of mice or spiders, fear of failure, fear of loss, fear of dying, or even of living: we deprive ourselves of a positive unfolding of our future. As form follows thought, so fear begets trauma. This form of fear is associated with emotional and material things in life.

The Action of the Remedy

The remedy brings a state of balance to over emotional fear. It does not overpower life-protecting caution, but releases us from the chains of futile fear. The person may still not like mice, spiders, heights, and so on but it is a more reasonable balanced caution of self-preservation rather than a neurotic over emotional fear.

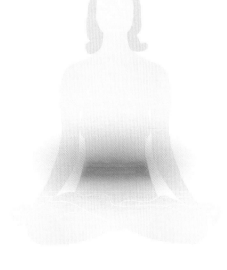

Tree

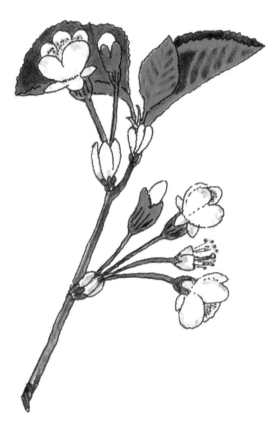

Qualities of the Tree

This tree often has a somewhat dishevelled appearance when growing wild. The early spring blossom bursts forth enthusiastically. In contrast, there is nothing disordered about the flowers. They are pure white blossoms, with five petals and long golden stamens, which bring a sense of peace and order to the whole tree.

Chakra Qualities

Sacral – *2nd Chakra*
Rainbow Colour – Orange

This energy quality of the Sacral Chakra keeps the emotional connection to the rational qualities of the Solar Plexus Chakra, establishing a sense of peace, order and harmony.

Positive Qualities

These people have a quality of calm steadfast courage. Their emotional balance and stability enable them to remain calm despite emotional and mental torment.

Negative State

Cherry plum is indicated for people who suffer from obsessive fears or delusions, which can lead to a fear of a nervous breakdown or even going insane. They feel as though they are sitting on an emotional pressure cooker: they can feel the pressure rising within them to the point where they feel they will explode and they can do nothing about it.

The Action of the Remedy

The remedy helps them to find an outlet for the pressure enabling them to regain emotional composure. They can then see the delusions for what they really are and begin to let go of them. The remedy helps people to regain their security by grounding them at a Base Chakra level and reconnect the Sacral Chakra to the higher Chakras so that they can find the inner wisdom and courage to face the real challenges in life and deal with them in a realistic, practical, emotionally balanced way.

Tree

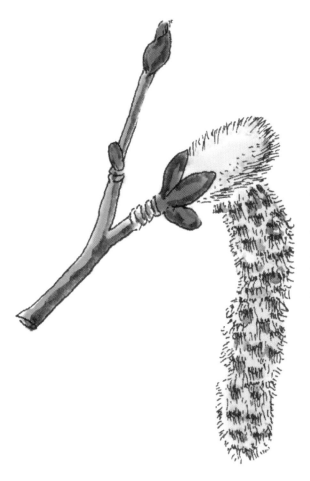

Qualities of the Tree

The long flattened stalks and rounded leaves cause this tree to appear to tremble in the slightest breeze as if it has a deep-seated trembling fear. However in sunlight the tremble becomes a shimmer with an ethereal quality.

Chakra Qualities

Sacral – *2nd Chakra*
Rainbow Colour – Orange

The quality of fearlessness, of trust in our higher self, and not being afraid to break new ground, with a strong connection to the groundedness of the Base Chakra.

Positive Qualities

These people love a challenge: they revel in the joy of life. They are warm, open, and friendly people.

Negative State

Aspen is indicated when a person's emotions are like the leaves on the aspen tree: they quiver at the least breath of wind. We have all been in places where we feel utterly vulnerable. A creepy, cold feeling comes over us, our hair stands on end and our skin develops goose bumps. This is the aspen fear. Those who suffer feel they have no protection from dark astral images and thought forms. Vague unreasoning fears of no known origin will suddenly creep over them, leaving them shaking with fear which they are unable to control. In this state, the Chakra is stuck open, which will allow any passing malevolent thought forms to enter.

The Action of the Remedy

The remedy will clear the shock in the system, or fear, which has overwhelmed the emotions and caused the Chakra to freeze in an open and vulnerable state. By calming the emotions, it will allow an easy gentle flow so that the Chakra can regain its normal function of opening to loved ones and closing defensively when negative energies are felt nearby.

Tree

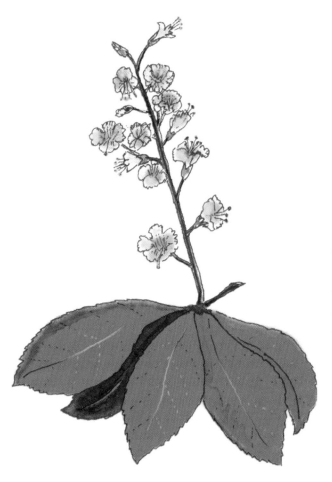

Qualities of the Tree

Similar in quality to the white chestnut in that they have beautiful conical shaped red flower groups, which from a distance resemble candles distributed throughout the tree. The red chestnut projects its personality outwards more so than its white counterpart.

Chakra Qualities

Sacral – *2nd Chakra*
Rainbow Colour – Orange

This quality connects us to a sense of inner calm and centeredness. It gives us the ability to allow others their path enabling us to focus on positive outcomes for all.

Positive Qualities

A joyous good-hearted person who projects positive energy to everyone they know. A mind that remains well balanced and positive even when under severe pressure.

Negative State

Red chestnut is a very interesting remedy, as it is not intended for the person who is suffering, but for the loved ones around the sufferer. How often do the loved ones project feelings of shock and sorrow when the person who they love is injured or ill? Just at the time when the patient needs positive love and help, the people caring for them are projecting emotions of fear and anger at the illness, shock and horror that the one they love is ill, and grief at the loss they fear they may experience. How often do parents sit up and worry if their teenage children are late home? If the child is feeling a little vulnerable, they can pick up on the projected negative energy, which of course will make them feel even worse. That is not to say that a balanced level of caution is not wise, it is the over-emotional projection of fear that is unwise.

The Action of the Remedy

The remedy enables those who need to help others, be they parents or nurses, doctors or therapists, to take a balanced emotional view. While they can be motivated by empathy for the sufferer and a desire to help, it will be a balanced emotion that will produce positive action. The desire to help will be carried out in a calm professional way, which is actually helpful, not a neurotic fearful way where the helper is of no use at all and in fact becomes part of the problem.

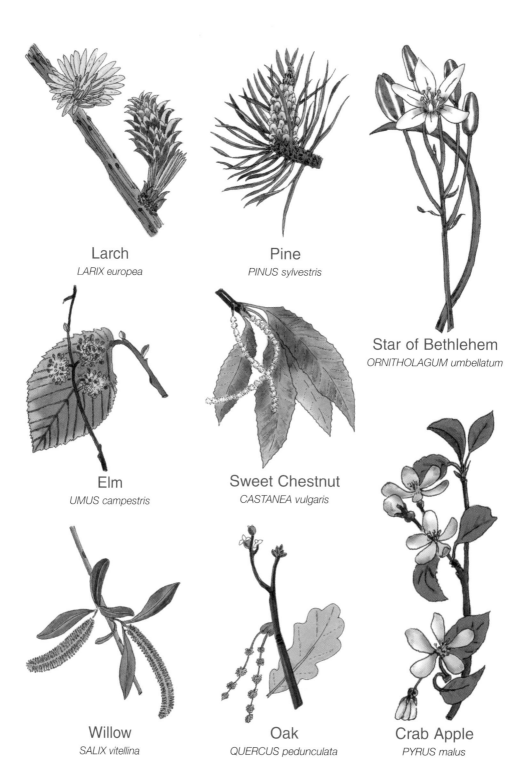

Larch
LARIX europea

Pine
PINUS sylvestris

Star of Bethlehem
ORNITHOLAGUM umbellatum

Elm
UMUS campestris

Sweet Chestnut
CASTANEA vulgaris

Willow
SALIX vitellina

Oak
QUERCUS pedunculata

Crab Apple
PYRUS malus

CHAPTER 11

Base Chakra and Remedies

Rainbow Colour Red

Energy Quality – Earth
1st Age – From Birth to 7 Years

Groundedness in the world, the material and the physical being, the drive to do, to be, and to survive, are basic to this Chakra. This is the turning point where our consciousness, having descended into matter, begins the return journey to the realms of spirit. This is where our attitudes to the physical world are manifested. When in balance, we achieve a groundedness in the world and a sense of belonging at a material and physical level. A free flow of energy leads to an inexhaustible force for work and the enormous mental and physical stability exhibited by martial arts experts.

We are comfortable and rejoice in our place in the world and in the world around us. It is our connection with mother earth and as such gives us access to the cleansing and protective properties available to us through the earth.

Imbalance manifests as obsessions with material gain: the aimless piling up of material possessions, gluttony, excessive drinking, sex without love, romance, or emotion, and an inability to find satisfaction from any quarter of life. Eventually, this leads to despondency and to despair as we never manage to connect the basic needs of our physical being to our spiritual consciousness, engendering primitive fears, exhaustion, and difficulty dealing with physical reality.

Remedy Group
Despondency, Despair

Remedies
Larch, Pine, Elm, Sweet Chestnut, Star of Bethlehem,
Willow, Oak, Crab Apple

Tree

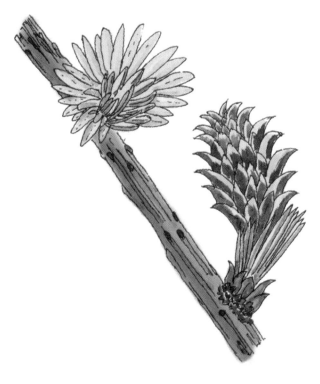

Qualities of the Tree

This is a tree on a mission as it is tuned into a short growing season. In its natural Northern European heartland, it is used to long winters and short summers. As a deciduous tree it has to re-establish its foliage each spring, and as a fast growing tree it demonstrates its ability to focus its energy and manifest its full potential.

Chakra Qualities

Base – *1st Chakra*
Rainbow Colour – Red

To begin to build we need good foundations. We cannot address our higher ideals until we feel secure at this level. When we are secure and grounded we can confidently open up to our higher energies in the confidence that we can achieve anything we wish.

Positive Qualities

These people are determined and capable. They have the will and drive to see things through to a successful outcome. They are the people who climb the every day mountains of life and who have the energy and the vision to cope with any challenge thrown up by life. They know what needs to be done and that if they do it now, a positive outcome is assured.

Negative State

Larch is indicated when people are always telling everyone about their problems. They will say, "It is just my luck – nothing works for me". They have no confidence in themselves and rob life of the opportunity to help them by only making indifferent effort. They have an air of procrastination, timidity and depression about them. They expect failure and life presents it to them in large measure. Others often see them as perfectly capable of managing their affairs if only they could get out from the negative cloud that follows them around everywhere. They just need a little sunshine in their lives.

The Action of the Remedy

In this state, the Chakra is just overbalanced by the pervasive clouds of negative energy that have accumulated around it. The remedy will balance the Chakra by raising its vibration to clear the negativity. This enables the energy from the higher Chakras to flow through. It also strengthens the connection from the Base Chakra to the Throat Chakra thereby firing the Base energy to manifest the intention that is held at the Throat level. The change in the person's state can be quite dramatic, as though someone has switched a light on within them.

Tree

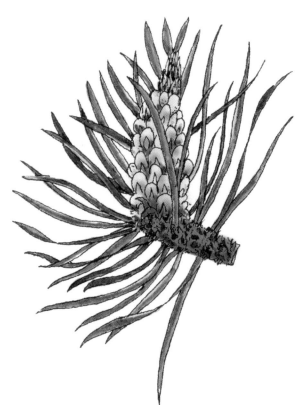

Qualities of the Tree

Everything about this tree reflects the clarity of its being. From the tall clean straight growth of the trunk and the sharp, thin, pointed needles to the clean, aromatic smell of the pine sap, the tree exudes a sense of cleanness and confidence.

Chakra Qualities

Base – *1st Chakra*
Rainbow Colour – Red

This connection at the Base Chakra cleanses and allows us to process experience without holding on or feeling responsible for all the problems around us. It is our ability to be the answer as opposed to being the problem.

Positive Qualities

These people are secure in the knowledge of their ability. They take responsibility (they have the ability to respond) without effort: in fact they enjoy the challenge and will enjoy the fruits of their efforts. While setting their sights high, they are connected to the bigger picture and see long-term achievements rather than short-term gains or losses.

Negative State

Pine is called for when people labour under a sense of guilt that eats away at the very foundations of their life, leaving them feeling totally insecure. They will condemn themselves and take the blame for things that are not their fault. This leads them to be over-conscientious, apologetic and embarrassingly humble. They never have a sense that anything they do can be good enough so they work harder to try to please. However the chasm of guilt becomes impossible to fill, so they are left physically drained by the effort they put in. They still feel guilty and depressed because in their eyes it was still not good enough. It is a state of self-absorption that is destroying to the soul.

The Action of the Remedy

The remedy helps to re-build the Base Chakra so that it releases that primal sense of guilt, almost at being born, so that it can feel good enough to be here. The Base Chakra energy needs to be grounded deep into the earth and know without question that it has the right to be here. This gives a tremendous feeling of stability and security that are the foundations from which a productive life can be built. This state enables the connection to the heart and to unconditional love, starting with oneself.

Tree

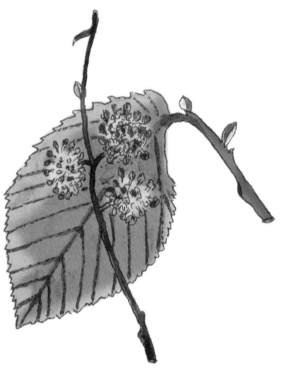

Qualities of the Tree

The elm tree has great strength but with a more delicate appearance than many large trees. It looks as though it is striving for greatness, and has a majesty that is combined with its delicate sensitivity.

Chakra Qualities

Base – *1st Chakra*
Rainbow Colour – Red

This is the quality of energy that connects us to the larger picture or vision of what we want to accomplish. This quality of energy gives us the strength and power to achieve our goals and visions in life.

Positive Qualities

These people are confident and self-assured decision-makers. They make good leaders because it is just part of their nature to take a positive attitude to responsibility. They know they have the skill and the ability to overcome any difficulties and ensure their intention is achieved.

Negative State

In this state people are temporarily overwhelmed by the weight of responsibility. The heavy load causes them to falter and feel they cannot carry on. When they are positive or at times when the load is slightly lighter, they manage perfectly well and even take a pride in the fact that they can cope easily. At these times they are affected by outside influences – sometimes with no bearing on the situation and these can be disabling even though they may not be directly relevant.

The Action of the Remedy

Occasionally a task is overwhelming and creates a lack of confidence until we reconnect to our Base Chakra strength and can continue. The remedy balances the over sensitivity to outer influences and gives a much-needed boost to the earth energy to keep us going. Often just one dose will be enough to get us back on our feet again, or at least allow us to re-gain our composure so that we can once again confidently tackle any task. Some people find it useful to take this remedy when they feel that the task is too difficult as it helps them to maintain balance and composure and both the strength and the vision to carry on.

Tree

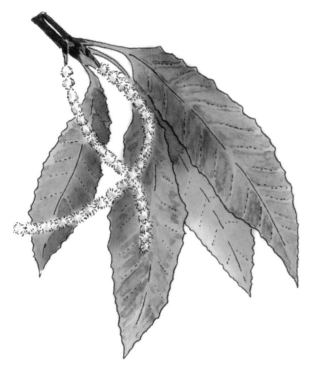

Qualities of the Tree

This is a tree of the most enduring stature. It is a tall and magnificent tree with the ability to live for hundreds of years. It has the capability of generating new growth out of what appears to be old and barren branches. When its golden catkins bloom profusely, they give the tree the appearance of having a golden aura.

Chakra Qualities

Base – *1st Chakra*
Rainbow Colour – Red

This level of energy has the quality of poise, self composure and confidence. When we are secure at this level, we ride the trials and losses of life in a philosophical way. We are not immune to grief, which is a natural and positive process, but have the security and faith drawn from the Crown level to survive any loss.

Positive Qualities

Is that very rare and very wonderful quality of faith which in spite of extreme anguish can, with absolute certainty, put its trust in divine providence to see it through. This quality is our connection to all that is and enables us to trust that whatever experiences we have in this incarnation, we are part of a bigger picture and as such are a manifestation of divine wisdom.

Negative State

Sweet chestnut is indicated for those times when everything seems lost: the experience is of absolute despondency and despair. The bottom has fallen out of our life. Literally the foundations seem destroyed, and there is nothing left to live for. It feels like the dark night of the soul: everywhere they look is darkness. This is the most extreme state, which Bach described. This state is brought on when the shock is so great that the consciousness has become locked in the Base Chakra. It has frozen, closed with fear and therefore is no longer able to allow the energy from the Crown Chakra and other higher Chakras to pass through.

The Action of the Remedy

The remedy helps to ease anxiety, and to release the 'white knuckle' grip on the fear. Once the person has begun to relax sufficiently to allow a trickle of energy through, they are able to get help from higher wisdom, which begins to send a glow of light into the darkness. Slowly, almost imperceptibly, the blackness begins to lift and the possibility of a solution begins to present itself. With each small increase in hope the condition eases, more energy from the Crown Chakra flows through and a greater level of hope and wisdom follow, until eventually the condition clears and a positive, hopeful view of life is re-established.

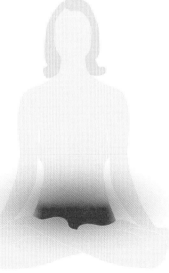

Flower

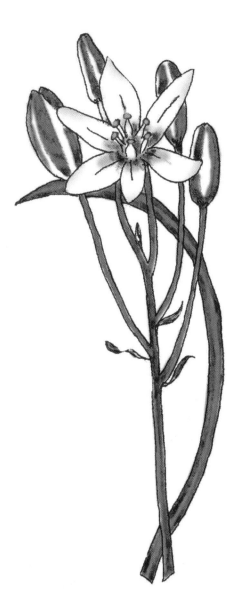

Qualities of the Flower

The first thing that strikes one about this flower is its six-petal formation. It epitomises a six-pointed Star of David with all the connotations of the balance between heaven and earth embodied in this flower's delicate shape.

Chakra Qualities

Base – *1st Chakra*
Rainbow Colour – Red

Throughout the Chakra system a constant flow between spiritual and physical takes place. The connection of Base Chakra through all levels to Crown Chakra and higher is the process that keeps 'body and soul together'.

Positive Qualities

This is found in those who have the ability to release the stress and tension caused by traumatic experiences. They retain strength and poise through difficult or shocking experiences and do not allow it to lock into their mind, their emotions or body but release the torment and shock and move on.

Negative State

Star of Bethlehem is the remedy for sudden shock that will, to the degree to which the shock is experienced, freeze the consciousness in the Base Chakra. This shock can sometimes get locked into the subconscious. The person may even feel that they have completely recovered only to find that they re-experience the trauma when in a similar situation or on the anniversary of the trauma. In cases of slight shock one dose of the remedy can bring about an almost miraculous recovery. More serious cases need to take the remedy for months or even years. In some cases it is useful to repeat the dosage on the anniversary of the shock.

The Action of the Remedy

The remedy eases and balances the energy of the Base Chakra to allow a free flow of energy from the Crown Chakra. It is really the disconnectedness from the Crown Chakra that causes the problem. The shock is merely the mechanism that brings the disconnectedness about. Conversely it is the re-establishment of the connection to the higher Chakras that solves the problem.

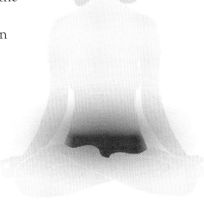

Tree

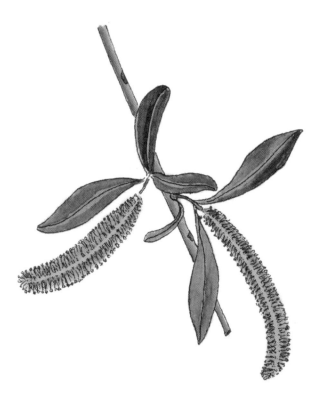

Qualities of the Tree

The willow has been of service to man throughout the ages. Its pliable versatile wood makes it useful for many purposes, from building to fencing, from charcoal for artists to basket weaving or making cricket bats. Over the years, it has been subjected to many forms of abuse, such as pollarding, but has a remarkable ability to re-grow and regenerate. This magnificent tree has an energy that is irrepressible.

Chakra Qualities

Base – *1st Chakra*
Rainbow Colour – Red

When all is said and done, what we make of our lives is up to us. At this level it is what we do – it is our ability to take responsibility for our actions and outcomes, readjusting to situations if things are not as we want. This is our will to be and our willingness to adapt.

Positive Qualities

This is seen in people who naturally attract the positive benefits of an optimistic personality. There is an old saying that "Good thoughts attract good things". People are naturally drawn to help the outgoing optimist whereas they avoid the pessimist.

Negative State

Willow is indicated when someone is impossible to please, always grumbling, spreading an air of despondency and gloom to those around them. They are bitter, bear grudges, sulk, blame others for their problems, and feel resentment that life should treat them so harshly. If they inherited or won a fortune they would complain that people only wanted them for what they could get out of them. They are humourless people who never know the true joy of giving. In this state, the person is totally cut off from the light and wisdom of the higher Chakras because their negativity blocks off the flow of higher energies through the Base Chakra. They destroy the base of their own lives and those of others because they are not able to see a way out.

The Action of the Remedy

The remedy helps to soften the harshness of the personality so that the higher energies can flow, bringing the energies of healing and wisdom to enable the person to see the true joy of life, of sharing and of being in harmony with others. It is sometimes said that a sad person cannot sing because there is no joy in him with which to make a song. A person in the negative willow state could never sing.

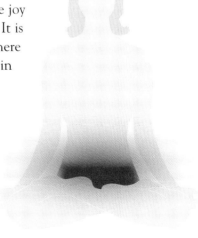

Tree

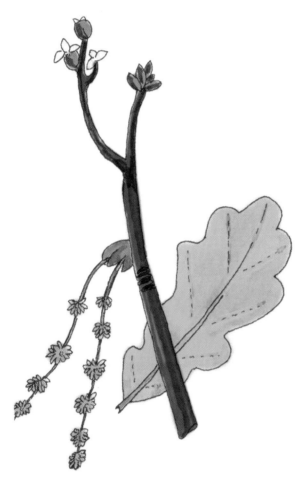

Qualities of the Tree

Sturdy and robust, its very wide girth renders it immovable, withstanding all sorts of battering from wind and storms. Its wide boughs and plentiful foliage protects and nurtures all around it. The oak will continue to live even when it is under great pressure or parts of it seem dead. Until one day caught unaware, the oak can no longer withstand the onslaught and it keels over. The oak's strength and solidity make it a popular building material.

Chakra Qualities

Base – *1st Chakra*
Rainbow Colour – Red

A strong Base connection gives us tremendous strength in the world and the ability to be a support to others in many ways. Within a balanced system this support is not abused, each person carries their own load so that no one is overburdened.

Positive Qualities

This is demonstrated in people who have the good common sense to know when to work and when to rest. They have the strength combined with wisdom to support others. They are grounded and can offer stability to those around them.

Negative State

The oak state is a more extreme version of the elm state. In this state, one has taken on too much or is being relied upon to too great a degree and is feeling the strain but defiantly would never admit it. They would willingly work until they drop rather than admit that they are finding things too much. This is not the work of a slave or a drudge but one who sees themselves as indispensable and would fear that the family may split up or the business may collapse if they do not carry on. Because they do not complain, others can grow to rely on them and ask them to take on an ever-increasing workload. 'Good old oak', never complaining, takes up the extra strain until the strain becomes too much, when to everyone's astonishment they break and collapse. This blocked oak energy is locked into the 'work ethic' of the Base Chakra to such an extent that it is unaware of the possibility of outside support. The negative oak state is a more extreme version of the negative elm state.

The Action of the Remedy

The remedy helps the person to get a more balanced view on life, to learn that it is not a weakness to bend a little and ask for help. They are often surprised when other people willingly and happily take on part of the burden, as they always imagined that they were the only ones that could cope.

Tree

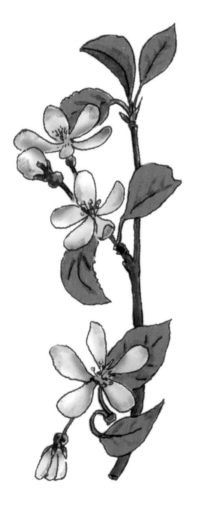

Qualities of the Tree

The wild crab apple is more bush-like than a domestic apple tree. Its name comes from the Norse 'Skarab' meaning scrubby. This seems the antipathy of the delicate pink tipped white flowers that adorn the bushy tree in spring like a cool, cleansing shower.

Chakra Qualities

Base – *1st Chakra*
Rainbow Colour – Red

All Chakras work together in harmonious unity although there are particular affinities between certain Chakras. Within the body, both the Crown Chakra and Base Chakra work together. High vibration energies from the Crown Chakra pour through the Base Chakra to enliven and cleanse any feelings of impurity. Drawing the higher energies down to clear negative thoughts and impressions through the Base Chakras earth connection, ensures that the two most effective and powerful cleansers, white light and mother earth, are available to us.

Positive Qualities

These people are in contact with and are constantly cleansed by the flow of energy from the higher Chakras. Their aura is clear and they look and feel as though they have a vibrancy and radiance about them that has a positive effect on everyone around them, which brightens the day for everyone they meet.

Negative State

In a negative crab apple state people feel in some way unclean. They may have a rash, a spot on the nose or simply have a feeling that there is something about them that is unwholesome and needs cleansing. This state is often accompanied by a feeling of general malaise because the Base Chakra has become slightly cut off from the energies of the Crown Chakra and feels the need for a good 'wash through' with the higher energies. The remedy is indicated when we have picked up a 'mood' or depression from those around us, something that does not really affect us but which we are trying to process, as healers sometimes do. Problems can also arise when a person takes a very narrow Base Chakra view of how the world should be, 'a place for everything and everything in its place' would be their motto. Anything that is out of place or not quite right can drive them to distraction.

The Action of the Remedy

The remedy will help to re-establish contact with the higher energies of the Crown Chakra. The purifying flow of higher energies will speed the vibration to the point where the Chakra 'glows' and no longer feels unclean. It helps to clear thought forms and worries from the aura. The increased flow of white light raises the energy to the point where petty concerns of self and obsessive physical perfection give way to more important values that can be taken up by the consciousness. This remedy is ideal for therapists to clear any residue of their clients negative energy. It should be taken along with walnut, which is both a mental protector and an aid to guiding clients through the changes they need to make.

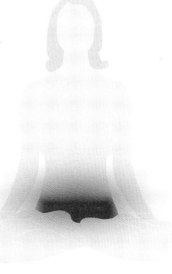

CHAPTER 12

Using the Remedies

Dr. Bach's remedies are made by one of two methods. Either 'The Sun Method', or 'The Boiling Method'. The former is used when imprinting the energy of fresh new blossoms. The latter is more often used for trees and buds where the energy is of a more robust quality or for remedies made at the beginning of the year when the sun is not strong. Both methods use heat to imprint the quality of the plant onto the water. This imprint is strongly held allowing the remedy to be used in most liquids, hot or cold.

Water: What is it and why is it used to make remedies?

About 65% of the weight of our body is water. All of the chemical reactions that take place in our body do so in water. We need water to live: without it we would shrivel and die. Water is a chemical compound of two simple elements: hydrogen and oxygen. When two atoms of hydrogen (H_2) combine with one atom of oxygen (O), the atom of oxygen is balanced between the two hydrogen atoms to form a water molecule (H_2O). The hydrogen in each water molecule forms a weak dipolar bond with the oxygen in other water molecules. In its liquid state, the bonds between the water molecules are constantly forming and breaking, causing intricate lacing patterns to be created and dissolved in the water. When we freeze water, we see these intricate lace patterns as ice crystals or snowflakes.

Scientists are now proving that water has a 'memory'. It can be imprinted with an energy pattern that can be detected. Crystal therapists and scientists know that crystals can carry information. So the intricate lattice crystals which form within liquid water can be impressed with an energy pattern.

Water is a living crystal – the remedies cause it to vibrate with flower energy.

Edward Bach developed his natural sensitivity to the point where he could feel the energy patterns on the dew of plants and flowers. He transferred these energy patterns to water by either the 'Sun Method' or the 'Boiling Method' and could feel the energy pattern in the water.

Dr. Bach used brandy as a 'preservative' to hold the energy pattern in the water. The remedy works best when drops are added to a glass of water. As the water dilutes the alcohol out, the remedy in the drops impregnates the crystal structure of the water, with the vibration of the remedy. The glass of water becomes a living crystal vibrating with flower energy. When we drink this water it impresses all of the water of our body with flower energy, which will in turn modify every chemical reaction that takes place in the water of our body. Because the remedy has a healing quality, this will emphasise all of the actions that are healing or building.

However, if illness is only at the stage of a disturbed energy in the aura and has not yet affected the physical body to cause disease, then we simply feel 'not quite ourselves'. Taking a remedy at this stage clears the disturbed mental or emotional pattern in the aura and therefore the disease never materialises in the physical body.

Making Stock Remedies

Dr. Bach described the process for making the remedies in his earlier books, by either of the following methods:

The Sun Method

A glass bowl is filled to within a couple of centimetres of the brim with pure water. Ideally this will be from a nearby spring whose water is noted for its healing qualities.

The bowl is set down in clear sunlight near the plant, and the best blooms floated on the water so as to cover the whole of the surface. After a while the water begins to bubble. This usually continues for two to four hours, depending on the strength of the sunlight: when the bubbling has stopped the water has taken on the energy of the flowers. The flowers are lifted off and the bottles are half filled with water. The bottles are topped up with brandy to preserve the remedies. These are stock bottles.

(You can experiment with garden flowers and float them on the water: watch the water begin to bubble. Do not take this as a remedy. Dr. Bach only used natural wild flowers as garden flowers are hybrid and comparatively very weak).

The Boiling Method

The selected parts of the plant, (buds, flowers, twigs, leafs) are placed into a pan of water, brought to the boil and simmered for 30 minutes. The liquid is drawn off, allowed to cool, and then bottled as in the Sun Method. To illustrate, if you have ever poured boiling water over a herbal tea bag, you have made a remedy by a method similar to the Boiling Method.

Using Remedies

We have found the following methods of taking or applying the remedies give good results:

1. Put two drops of the remedy into a glass of pure water, and sip slowly.
2. Purchase dropper bottles from the chemist, nearly fill with water, and add two drops of remedy from the stock bottle. Take as drops onto the tongue or add to a teaspoon full of water. To preserve this remedy add a teaspoon of brandy. When dealing with recovering alcoholics use a teaspoon of vinegar as a preservative.
3. Apply as a compress directly to a chakra.
4. Drops of remedy can also be taken by adding them to any non-alcoholic drink, tea, coffee, fruit juices, soups, etc. Bach remedies are unaffected by heat, because either the heat of the sun or boiling is used to make the remedies.
5. Add the remedies to a small glass of water; drink half of the water whilst settling down to sleep and the other half first thing in the morning. This system enables you to ensure you have at least two 'doses' a day. For sleep problems, an appropriately identified remedy taken in this way will be of great benefit.
6. When treating babies. If the mother is breast-feeding she can take the remedy and the baby will receive it through her milk. When bottle-feeding, add a drop of remedy to the feed or add a couple of drops to baby's bath water.
7. Remedies added to bath water give a wonderfully relaxing bath. They are unaffected by aromatic oils or soaps.
8. For specific areas of the body, say a swollen knee, low back, painful neck, or whatever, a compress can be very useful. To make a compress, take a shallow dish, add water that is comfortably warm to the touch, add remedies to the water, soak a cloth or bandage in the water, wring out the excess water and apply to the part to be treated. Hold in place with a bandage.
9. To treat animals, add the remedies to their drinking water.
10. To treat plants, add the remedies to the water in a watering can.

In cases of great distress, the remedy may be taken every few minutes until there is an improvement: in severe cases, say every half hour. Be guided by the need of the patient and give as often as needed. When dealing with a deep-rooted problem, it may be necessary to treat for weeks or months. In cases of severe shock, it can be useful to treat on the anniversary of the shock until it has completely cleared out of the system.

Specific Tips for Therapists

As therapists you may, like us, never have time to make remedies for yourselves. We use remedies made by the main remedy suppliers.

1. Acupuncturists and kinesiologists. Add the remedies to water, soak a small piece of cotton wool and apply to an acupuncture point. Hold in place with surgical tape. Or clear a meridian by running along the meridian with the soaked cotton wool.
2. Reflexologists. Apply to reflex points or clear along zones, as above.
3. Place a small amount of massage oil in a dish, add the remedies, and mix. This can be a little difficult, as oil and water do not mix easily. Apply to the part to be treated.
4. To clean the energy in a treatment room, purchase a plant sprayer from a garden shop. Nearly fill the sprayer with water, add remedies, turn the sprayer nozzle onto fine mist and spray the room. Be particularly aware of corners as the energy easily stagnates there.
5. Recommend that clients take as soon as possible after surgery, to clear the shock of the operation and the anaesthetic out of the system.
6. For protection when treating clients who have a negative mental state, take walnut as a mental protector and crab apple to clear out any negative energy that you inadvertently picked up during the treatment.

CHAPTER 13

Journal Keeping with the Remedies

As the inspiration for this book grew out of journal keeping, we felt it would not be complete without at least an introduction to this incredibly fulfilling self-development tool.

It is important to realise that we are all on a journey, and part of that journey is finding space to allow growth and healing through change. These changes are a natural part of moving freely along life's path. Resistance to change holds us back and interrupts our smooth passage along our way. Those who work with journal keeping and the Bach remedies will find that their resistances dissolve more easily allowing things in their lives that need to change to be able to do so. We cannot honour another person's journey without understanding that they too are on a path. Change is something they will accept in their own time, when they will begin to release the negative emotions and thought patterns that have hitherto obstructed their path.

We must be in touch with our own weaknesses, needs, feelings and fears, as well as capitalising on our strengths and opportunities. Without this understanding we cannot forge our own path or develop the empathy and patience needed to support others through their own growth and development.

With this in mind, we introduce you to journal keeping, giving you the opportunity to observe your own path. You can then use the Bach remedies to rebalance or re-pattern negative attitudes or emotions, working towards positive strengths or 'virtues' as Dr. Bach called them.

To experience this process for yourself, try this simple game. Write down the question: "How do I feel?" and then write down your answer. Quite often people only pay attention to their feelings when something wonderful or alternatively something dreadful happens. It is a little like only eating food that is gourmet or burnt. There are many subtle tones to our emotions that are easily missed. When we are in touch with them, we experience these many subtleties, thereby enhancing the quality of our life.

Then write down the question: "What do I want?" and then your answer. In fairy stories, when a person is given three wishes, they are either wasted, or the outcome is disastrous. Although people often complain about what is wrong with their lives, they are experts on what they don't want, but they have never addressed the simple question: "If I could have what I want, what would it be?"

Honest answers to these two questions can put you in touch with depths of feeling and of directions you want to take in life that will make enormous improvements to the quality of your life.

When we work with this process, the challenge is to find a way to achieve: 'What we want'. To do this, we must take appropriate action, neither too much nor too little, appropriate to the challenge. We may do this in the company of others as say, dancing, or we may need to act alone, as when walking a mountain path. In each case, we may choose a remedy or several remedies to help us move forward.

For instance, to act appropriately we need to consider what our path might be. Wild oat can be particularly helpful here. When we have chosen a goal that our heart desires, there arises an inevitable tension between what we are and where we are right now, and the path or course of action we need to follow to get to where we want to be. To face this fear, aspen might be useful. We now need to choose a line of action from the many opportunities or challenges we face: scleranthus can be helpful here to enable us to choose a path. Then other remedies will come into play depending on whether the reluctance to move forward comes from a harking back to the past: "It was easier then" or "If only I had made better use of my opportunities". Here, honeysuckle will be helpful. Perhaps there are lots of plans and ideas but difficulty 'getting your head out of the clouds' and doing something practical, then clematis will help. If you feel a bit flat and can't get started, try hornbeam.

By working with our heart-felt desires and ambitions in the journal, we identify blocks to the flow of energy in our lives. Then those remedies that we need to help us work through the blocks become clearer. At any time that we are working through transitions in our lives or dealing with changing circumstances then walnut will help us to move through the changes with poise and a positive outlook.

For those of you who wish to make journal keeping a part of your own journey, a more detailed and in depth look at your life is needed. To help you to do this we offer the following suggestions but always remember your journal is about you, so ultimately the way you keep it will be the way that most suits you. Take what is useful from the following and try it.

1. **Do not use loose-leaf paper**
   Use a book to ensure that everything stays together. If in a moment of inspiration you write on the back of an envelope, wrapping paper or any other scrap of available paper you can either paste or tape it into your book later. It is a good idea to keep these scraps of paper, as they will help to remind you of the emotions that were going through your mind and body at the time you wrote them.

2. **Date every entry**
   It may not seem very important to you as you pour your heart out on to the page, but it will be of enormous importance when the event has passed and you want to see it in its place, without the emotional investment you had in it.

3. **Only enter your journal two or three times per week**
   It is important that your journal is not a chore. However it sometimes helps to get started by setting a routine of say twice a week. That doesn't mean that if you feel moved to, you can't pick it up in the meantime and work in it.

4. **Write about how you feel**
   Do not just itemise whom you met and what happened. The world may have just gone through the most dramatic events imaginable. If you want to write about them, try to write how you feel about them. On the other hand if you prefer to write about how it feels to have seen an old friend or about raindrops on a flower, then do. Your journal is about you, so leave it to the newspapers to write about the world.

5. **Write about what you want**
   As we grow up we are taught in many different ways: 'I want never gets'. Many of our ideas are put down or ridiculed by others and to be accepted we change our thought patterns to fit what seems to be required by our 'judges'. When we get in touch with what we really want and open ourselves to accepting it, we find the changes we desire manifest seemingly effortlessly.

6. **Do not edit what you write**
   Just let it pour onto the page as it comes. I have often been writing something and decided it was rubbish and needed altering. On the occasions when I have gone back and altered it before continuing, it has in fact turned out to be rubbish. When I have had the courage to just continue and trust, I have been wonderfully surprised by the quality and content of the finished piece.

7. **Do not allow anyone to read your journal**
   It is a private place where you can be completely yourself. Always know when you write, that what you write is for you alone, and that you need never be inhibited about what you feel or how you express yourself. It will be your truth about you with all of its heights, depths and inconsistencies. If you stay really true to yourself, you will find that you are not the simple person you may think you are, but a many faceted individual where the parts sometimes love and sometimes conflict with each other. When you know that, you will also know that everyone else in the world is also a mass of loving and conflicting drives. It can take time, a little love, respect and trust in you, to get to that point. However the fulfilment we gain by travelling the path is well worth the effort.

Our reason for moving away from the traditional method of looking at the remedies, which focuses on the negative states to be treated was to look more to the positive aspects of the remedies. When we encourage students to use them in conjunction with journal keeping as a self-development tool, they need to look away from the negative state they are experiencing, and towards the positive outcome they desire. As they do this they begin to change, grow and develop. They go through an experiential growth process, similar in its pattern but not in its detail to that which can be seen in any person who makes profound and positive changes in their lives.

Often this process begins with discontentment with present circumstances, but continuing with the search for a new direction to bring about the desired improvements in life. Ultimately they begin to realise that peace and contentment come from the simplicity of life, not the turmoil of the mind. In this process the person has to face and deal with new challenges, with hope fulfilled and disappointments experienced. Continually reassessing their situation and learning to allow change to be able to move forward in the flow of life. Eventually understanding that true inner power comes from a calm and peaceful connection to their source.

While we were looking at Edward Bach's life, we were struck by how he was on his own developmental path and how he struggled with ideas and change. First as a doctor, then a bacteriologist and researcher, then working with homoeopathy until finally finding the very powerful simplicity he sought in the healing herbs of the fields, hedgerows and meadows.

Quick Reference to Remedies

Quick Reference to Remedies in Alphabetical Order

Some Suppliers of Remedies, Books, Audio Tapes and Posters

Ainsworths Essences

36. New Cavendish Street
London
W1G 8UF
Send stamped addressed envelope for
free Quick Guide to Bach Remedies
Tel.: +44 (0) 207 486 4313
E-mail: London@ainsworths.com
Web: www.ainsworths.com

Also certified courses at:
The Bach Flower
Educational Foundation

42. Welbeck Street
London, W1
Tel.: +44 (0) 207 935 5330
Ainsworths are founder members of
The British Association of Flower
Essence Producers (BAFEP), an
association for Bach Flower and other
essence producers, which sets and
maintains the highest standards and
monitors Government regulatory
requirements.

International Flower
Essence Repertoire

Achamore House
Isle of Gigha
Argyle & Bute
PA41 7AD, Scotland
Tel.: +44 (0) 1583 505385
E-mail: flower@atlas.co.uk
Web: www.ifer.co.uk
For information on a wide range of
international flower essences.

Healing Herbs Ltd.

P.O. Box 65
Hereford
HR2 0DX, UK
Tel.: +44 (0) 1873 890218
Fax.: +44 (0) 1873 890314
Web: www.healingherbs.co.uk
For remedies, books, tapes and posters.

Dr. Edward Bach Centre

Mount Vernon
Brightwell-cum-Sotwell
Wallingford, Oxon, UK
OX10 0PZ, UK
Tel.: +44 (0) 1491 834678
Web: www.bachcentre.com
For remedies, books, tapes and posters.

The Bach Remedies and the Chakras

Chakra	Positive Quality	Positive States of Each Remedy
CROWN Violet	Universal. Connected to the divine.	Natural poise, grace and dignity. Good listeners. Helpful, wise counsellors. Patient. Content to let the will of heaven unfold. Understanding of others. Draws strength from the divine. Natural inner strength. Shares the burden of others.
BROW Indigo	Intuitive. Clear slighted. The connection between the mind and higher wisdom.	The selfless server. Gives space to others to allow their growth. Calm and steadfast. Accepting of others' opinions. A good listener. Tolerant and kind. Encourages others to excel at their own pace. Strong wise leader. Helpful. Teaches and guides others. Emphatic. Flexible. Tolerant while remaining balanced.
THROAT Blue ETHER	Divine will. Healing and communication. The connection to your life path.	Grounded yet with a lively interest in life. Inspired yet capable of building the vision. Retains wisdom from past experiences; no wallowing in nostalgia. Lives in the swim of life. Grasps the power and joy of the moment. A calm resolute focus on the vision. Strength of mind. Calm, focused thoughts. Unaffected by outside influences. Constant stability and joy. Unshakeable inner serenity. Keen observer of life. Learns from mistakes. Absorbs information.
HEART Green AIR	Transformation and balance. The ability to act from the heart. Unconditional love.	A genuine optimist. Heartfelt warmth and humour. Fearless in adversity. Strong character. Knows when to give and when to be firm. Serves from the heart. Strength with balance. Has the strength to handle changing circumstances. Warm hearted. Loving. Generous. Tolerant of others.
SOLAR PLEXUS Yellow FIRE	Instinctive. Thinking and feeling. Clarity. Knowing what to do or build.	Decisive. Firm resolve. Acts correctly on intuitive impulse. Well balanced. Resolute action. Knows what action to take. Trusts intuition. Faces adversity courageously. Brushes aside setbacks. Sees task completed. Convictions that outcomes will be positive. Has great faith. Radiates joy and vitality. Inner strength. Bright joyous outlook. Vibrant energy. Enjoys a challenge. Clear vision of the future. Recognises the right path. Ambitious.
SACRAL Orange WATER	Emotions. Creativity and sexuality. The joy of giving and receiving.	Bravery. Heroism. Steadfastness. The courage to take action. Gentle courage. Balance. Serenity. Clear unworried mind. Remains calm despite mental and physical torment. Calm steadfast courage. Revels in the joy of life. Loves challenge and adventure. Projects positive energy to all. Well balanced mind.
BASE Red EARTH	The will to live. The drive to act and manifest things at a spiritual level.	Has the will to see things through. Determined and capable. Takes responsibility with joy and true humility. Secure in one's ability. Positive attitude to responsibilities. Confident, self-assured leader and decision-maker. In spite of extreme anguish can trust divine providence to see them through. Retains strength and poise through the torment of shock and anguish. Attracts the positive benefits of an optimistic personality. Strength combined with wisdom to support others. Knows when to work/rest. In contact with and cleansed by the flow of higher energy.

Remedy Group	Remedy	Negative States of Each Remedy
LONELINESS. Disconnected from the divine.	Water Violet Impatiens Heather	Aloof. Arrogant. Condescending. Impatient. Nervous irritability. Emotionally draining.
OVERCARE FOR THE WELFARE OF OTHERS. Projecting out into the world.	Chicory Vervain Beech Vine Rock Water	Demands attention. Argumentative. Forcefully opinionated. Dominating. Critical. Harsh authoritarian. Arrogant. Bossy. Manipulative. Stiff personality. Narrow minded.
LACK OF INTEREST IN PRESENT CIRCUMSTANCES. Needs to be in THE NOW.	Clematis Honeysuckle Wild Rose Olive White Chestnut Mustard Chestnut Bud	Air head. Daydreamer. Lives in the past. Gives up on life. 'No point trying'. Total fatigue of mind and body. Revolving thoughts. Endless mind chatter. Depression that descends and clears suddenly. Repeats mistakes. Never learning.
OVERSENSITIVITY TO INFLUENCES AND IDEAS. Unable to transmute energy due to lack of balance.	Agrimony Centaury Walnut Holly	Puts on a brave face. Servile. Easily dominated by others. Unbalanced by life's changes. Bitter. Gnarled. Angry.
UNCERTAINTY. No clear vision. Disconnected from the Throat Chakra.	Cerato Scleranthus Gentian Gorse Hornbeam Wild Oat	Indecisive. Weak willed. Vacillation, this or that? Easily discouraged. Fire of vitality extinguished. Needs a boost. Just a bit low. Cannot see the big vision.
FEAR. Needs to be anchored to the Heart Chakra. Needs courage.	Rock Rose Mimulus Cherry Plum Aspen Red Chestnut	Panic stricken. Frozen. Emotional or irrational known fear. Feels pressurised. Wants to lash out. Trembles with fear or dread. Projects fear and negativity.
DESPONDENCY AND DESPAIR. Lost in the material world. Disconnected from the Crown Chakra.	Larch Pine Elm Sweet Chestnut Star of Bethlehem Willow Oak Crab Apple	Expects failure. Fears success. Blames self without reason. Temporary loss of confidence. Feels all is lost. Extreme anguish. Locked in profound shock. Poor me. Weeping. Resentful. Supports everyone, except self. Feels mentally and physically unclean.

Bibliography

Anderson, M.: 1975. *Colour Healing Chromatherapy: How it Works.* Thorsons, London.

Anderson, M.: 1990. *Colour Therapy: The Application of Colour for Healing Diagnosis and Well-being.* The Aquarian Publishing, UK.

Bach, Dr. E.: 1994. *Collected Writings of Edward Bach.* Ashgrove Publishing, UK.

Bach, Dr. E.: 1996. *Heal Thyself: Explanation of the Real Cause and Cure of Disease.* C. W. Daniel, Woodbridge, UK.

Bach, Dr. E.: 2002. *The Twelve Healers and Other Remedies.* Pilgrims Publishing.

Baker, Dr. D. M.: 1978. *Esoteric Healing: Flower Remedies and Medical Astrology,* v.3. Baker Publications.

Barnard, J.: 2000. *A Guide to the Bach Flower Remedies.* C. W. Daniel, Woodbridge, UK.

Barnard, J.: 1987. *Patterns of Life Force.* Flower Remedy Programme.

Barnard, J., and Barnard, M.: 1994. *The Healing Herbs of Edward Bach: Illustrated Guide to the Flower Remedies.* Ashgrove Publishing, UK.

Bricknell, C. (Ed.): 1989. *RHS Encyclopaedia of Flowers and Plants.* Dorling Kindersley, London.

Davidson, J. 1988. *The Web of Life.* C. W. Daniel, Woodbridge, UK.

Genders, R. (Ed.). 1975. *Pear's Encyclopaedia of Gardening.* Mayflower.

Rainer, T.: 1980. *The New Diary: How to Use a Journal for Self-guidance and Expanded Creativity.* Angus and Robertson.

Reader's Digest. 1981. *Field Guide to Trees and Shrubs of Britain.* Reader's Digest, Devon, UK.

Reader's Digest. 2001. *Field Guide to the Wild Flowers of Britain.* Reader's Digest, Devon, UK.

Reader's Digest. 1984. *Guide to Creative Gardening.* Reader's Digest, Devon, UK.

Rendal, P.: 1990. *Understanding the Chakras: Discovering and Using the Energy of Your Seven Vital Force Centres.* Harper Collins, London.

Scheffer, M.: 1998. *Bach Flower Therapy: The Complete Approach.* Harper Collins, London.

Stone, R.: 1986. *Health Building: The Conscious Art of Living Well.* CRCS Publications, USA.

Tompkins, C. P.: 1974. *The Secret Life of Plants.* Harper Collins, London.

Weeks, N.: 1940. *The Medical Discoveries of Edward Bach, Physician.* C. W. Daniel, Woodbridge, UK.

White, R.: 1993. *Working With Your Chakras.* Piatkus, London.

Wills, P.: 1993. *Colour Therapy: The Use of Colour for Health and Healing.* Element, UK.